HOW TO USE TI
IN AN EMERGᴇ...

1.

Look up the poison in the Index at the back of the book (p. 107). All substances are listed by the kind of product they are. (Therefore, for Handy Andy or Ajax, for example, look up **Cleaners.**)

2.

Turn to the page indicated for information on symptoms and treatment. Please note that T.R. means Toxicity Rating — each substance is given a rating which tells you how poisonous it is. The scale is explained on p. 63.

3.

Treat the poisoning as suggested. Instructions on how to induce vomiting etc. are on p. 60.

4.

Don't forget there is a Poison Information Centre in all capital cities and their telephone number is listed with the emergency numbers. If you have ANY doubts, ALWAYS ring rather than hope you are doing the right thing.

HELEN McCAUGHEY

IS IT

POISONOUS?

Poisoning Prevention and First Aid

A Lifesaving Manual

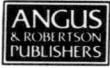

ANGUS
& ROBERTSON
PUBLISHERS

To Gerald Stone—friend and urger.

ANGUS & ROBERTSON PUBLISHERS

Unit 4, Eden Park, 31 Waterloo Road,
North Ryde, NSW, Australia 2113, and
16 Golden Square, London W1R 4BN,
United Kingdom

First published in Australia
by Angus & Robertson Publishers in 1976
Revised edition 1980
Reprinted 1984
This paperbound edition 1987
Reprinted 1987

© Helen McCaughey 1976

National Library of Australia
Cataloguing-in-publication data

McCaughey, Helen.
  Is it poisonous?

  Rev. ed.
  ISBN 0 207 15558 5 (pbk.).

  1. Poisons — Safety measures. 2. Poisoning —
  Treatment. I. Title.
615.9'05

Printed in Singapore

ACKNOWLEDGMENTS
I would like to thank Dr Margaret Burgess for her invaluable help with the section on drug-induced effects on the foetus and breastfed baby, Dr John Woolnough for his permission to print details of his superb childproof cupboard invention, Dr Bob Webb for help with the Drug Abuse section and Dr John Tomkins for the unique information he supplied for the chapter on bites and stings. I would particularly like to thank Bruce McDonald and the staff of the Poison Information Centre at the Royal Children's Hospital in Melbourne for their advice and help in revising the third edition.

NOTE
Helen McCaughey was a professional employee of the Poisons Information Centre, Sydney, New South Wales. This book was written by her in her private capacity and no official support or endorsement by the centre is intended or inferred.

AUTHOR'S NOTE TO THE SECOND EDITION
I have made some minor changes to the text, but the major improvement to this edition is the addition of a comprehensive Index of substances commonly swallowed by accident (or by design, as in the case of curious children and attempted suicides). This Index should help you to locate quickly the information you need in an emergency. So. . .

FOREWORD

Helen McCaughey's very practical and particularly lucid textbook reflects her very wide experience of the innumerable problems associated with the prevention and treatment of various forms of accidental poisoning during infancy and childhood and also includes valuable information on poisoning in adult life, food and plant poisoning, bites and stings, ingested and inhaled foreign bodies and certain significant hazards associated with drug ingestion during pregnancy and lactation.

The extremely large number of potentially toxic substances which may be swallowed by children in or outside their homes is increasing at an alarming rate and there is an obvious need for full and adequate advice about the prevention and treatment of all forms of accidental poisoning during childhood. Accurate information about the incidence of poisoning amongst Australian children would seem to be difficult to obtain but the number of infants and children admitted to the Royal Alexandra Hospital for Children over the past 20 years because of poisoning has increased by more than 300 per cent while the overall admissions have increased by only 20 per cent.

In March 1966 the Royal Alexandra Hospital for Children, prompted by the obvious and rapid increase in the incidence of poisoning during childhood, established New South Wales' first Poisons Information Centre with the main object of providing immediate advice and help to all sections of the community and more particularly to parents and to members of the medical, pharmaceutical and nursing professions.

In December 1967 Helen McCaughey was appointed director of this centre and for the next three years answered innumerable urgent questions from distressed parents and guardians and from medical practitioners, pharmacists and nurses about poisoning in its many and different forms. Since her retirement from the directorship of this unit she has continued her work in this particular field by serving as a part-time member of Sydney's after-hours Poisons

Information Centre, as a "drug educator" on the staff of the Health Commission of New South Wales, and in 1974 was responsible for writing the Poisons Section of the *Australian Pharmaceutical Formulary.*

Lorimer Dods
Emeritus Professor of Child Health
University of Sydney
1976

CONTENTS

x

INTRODUCTION

To many people, and particularly to mothers of young children, the prospect of having to deal with an accidental poisoning is extremely frightening. The fear is intensified by an often vague and limited knowledge on the subject of poison. Which substances are dangerous, and which harmless or just mildly distressing when swallowed? When should vomiting be induced, and when should it be prevented?

In this book I have attempted to answer questions like these, and to dispel some of the fear and panic which surrounds the whole question of poisoning.

The most important part of the book is the Poison List, which lists all the substances, from acids to zinc cream, which in my experience are most commonly sampled by children (experimentally) and by adults (accidentally). The List has been designed as a quick reference, giving information on how poisonous each substance is, first symptoms after it has been swallowed, inhaled, or splashed on to the skin or in the eye, and first aid. Because of their diversity Garden Chemicals have been given a chapter of their own, and first aid and symptom information for specific chemicals may be found in chart form in this chapter. Poisonous plants, because they are so numerous and their toxicity so variable, have also been dealt with in a separate chapter. See the alphabetical list of plants for first aid instructions.

I have also included some general chapters on food poisoning, garden chemicals, poisonous plants, poisoning of pets, bites and stings, swallowed objects and choking, and drug abuse. The three last topics are, I suppose, not conventionally thought of as types of poisoning. I have included the chapters because of the large number of inquiries I have received at the Poisons Information Centre concerning these subjects.

The book also includes general chapters on first aid and poison prevention.

Obviously, prevention is better than cure, and where possible everyone would like to avoid the panic and upset which even a mild poisoning scare causes. Prevention is not always possible, but understanding when and why poisonings are likely to occur helps a great deal. Child poisoning and accidental adult poisoning have in general quite different patterns and characteristics. A general discussion of each will make this clear.

CHILD POISONING

If you have a child who has never eaten anything that he shouldn't — not a snail, a dirty old dog's bone, a couple of oral contraceptive tablets, the felt nose from his favourite teddy or some caps from his brother's capgun — then you are fussing too much over his safety. It is all just part of learning the difference between food and everything else. We aren't born with the talent, it must be learned, and as with everything else your child will learn by making mistakes. Most of the episodes of accidental ingestion in childhood upset the parent far more than the child. All the panic is very often a waste of energy, only helping to make the episode a good story to tell your friends after it's all over.

It's not a bad idea to let the child gulp a few nasty tasting things from kitchen cupboards rather than to keep everything out of reach. If you refer to the Index you will be able to pick out a few safe things that taste awful. Plenty of kitchen items such as detergent, window cleaner and laundry blue, can be left down in available cupboards. Familiarity breeds contempt and conversely the things you do lock up gain great interest value. Children will go to no end of trouble to get to the forbidden fruit. On top of the refrigerator is not good enough — high cupboards for an ingenious two–year–old mean nothing except a more desirable quarry. Ideally a childproof cupboard (as described and illustrated in the Poison Prevention chapter) should be put in so that you can keep all your problem bottles and cans in one handy place.

I emphasise "handy" because I do believe that unless your cupboard is very conveniently placed you will put the tablets or the kerosene down "for just a second" after use instead of returning them to their rightful place immediately and zap — your two–year–old will have done it again. How often have I heard that story!

The old adage that things go wrong at the most awkward times has some logic behind it. Frequently I hear poisoning stories involving one of the following reasons: "We were visiting"; "We were going on holidays the next day"; "I was cleaning out the cupboard"; "Grandmother was staying with us"; "One of the children was sick". When circumstances around the house are not as normal, when the daily humdrum routine has been interrupted and some special event is occurring, that is when your concentration on child safety wavers, and the disasters occur.

I vividly remember one case where the family was thrown into confusion by a child who had managed to make a cocktail of antiseptic, nasal spray, nasal drops, burn cream, suppositories for constipation, antihistamine tablets, antibiotic tablets and blood pressure tablets. She ate some of this gluey, colourful mess but with rapid treatment survived unscathed. The poisoning occurred because while a sick member of the family was being dosed the medicine cabinet, loaded with poisons and usually locked, was left open.

In another case an overseas trip was put off only hours before the family was to board the boat — tablets which had never been available before were left out, and eaten by a child.

Don't feel too guilty if accidents like this occur, but do your best to avoid them. If your child eats anything it shouldn't, do something about it **immediately**. Never wait to see if symptoms develop. On the other hand, panic will do no good at all. Be reassured that in most cases so long as you get medical help or advice quickly, everything will be all right. The Index at the back of this book will refer you to advice on first aid measures to take while you are waiting. If you are not sure what has been taken, or cannot find the substance taken in the Index, give milk while you are waiting for medical help — dilution of the poison is often a good idea, and never a bad one.

The most commonly swallowed products are the things which most commonly occur about the house. Detergent is usually number one, followed by painkilling tablets, toilet deodorant blocks, cough mixtures, oral contraceptives and household cleaners. When a new floor polish or fly spray comes on to the market the Poisons Information Centre hears about it very quickly — and the number of children eating it reflects how well it is penetrating the market. Perhaps market researchers should interview us to help them with their investigations!

It is interesting to note the seasonal variations in poisoning cases. In winter there is always a rash of antibiotic and cough mixture cases and in summer the Poisons Information Centre receives incessant calls about swimming pool chemicals and sunburn cream.

Luckily, the most commonly ingested products aren't very poisonous and with rapid treatment children who have eaten them rarely need hospital attention.

For all details about individual substances — those that are particularly dangerous and those that can be left about without danger — read quickly through the Poison List at the back of the book. Special attention should be given to the dangerous chemicals that must be kept out of reach, such as antidepressant tablets, iron tablets, asthma tablets or suppositories with aminophylline in them, camphorated oil, all kerosene, turps and petrol-like things, liquid furniture polish, liquid fly spray, ant killers, oven and drain cleaners, soldering fluxes containing zinc chloride, all pesticides, digoxin heart tablets and aspirin, to name a few. Aspirin is of particular danger in small children when the dosage on the label is not strictly adhered to, and is better not used at all in children under three years old.

ACCIDENTAL ADULT POISONING

The reasons for the accidental poisoning of adults come under a very few headings. These specific areas of misuse recur with monotonous regularity and often with disastrous results.

Storage of poisons in food containers

Two old ladies who were normally abstemious decided to celebrate the 74th birthday of one of them early on a Tuesday morning by opening a bottle of sweet sparkling wine. The bottle had been about for ages and was rusty around the cork, but not wanting to seem ungrateful the birthday girl gulped two mouthfuls — and said not a word. The hostess realised there was a mistake before she tasted hers but her friend became unconscious from an enormous dose of dieldrin, a pesticide, in 15 minutes. Very active therapy saved her, but only just.

Others have been less lucky. The situation has often arisen because a chemical used at work was thought to be a good product, and a little was decanted off in a drink bottle to use at home. Chlordane, another pesticide, goes milk coloured when diluted and so very often a milk bottle is chosen as a container. Paraquat, a weedkiller, has killed four people to my personal knowledge because it has a similar colour to cola and was gulped accordingly. Condy's crystals when dissolved are also cola coloured and too often find their way into cola bottles. Even strong arsenic solution isn't vastly different from whisky and caused the death of a man who had just returned from his wife's funeral.

Not reading the label

Nobody reads labels until something goes wrong — I don't know why, but this seems to be a universal shortcoming. So people often eat and drink things not meant for consumption, and take large quantities of medicine meant to be measured in small doses.

Five teaspoonfuls (instead of mls) of antibiotic every six hours will use up your medicine too quickly, or have even more disastrous effects. One infirm elderly gentleman took a tablespoonful of tablets, luckily vitamins, and only when his daughter discovered him 10 minutes later, still at it, did she stop him and discover that 82 tablets covered a tablespoon.

Pesticides are a classic source of poisoning because labels aren't read. The case histories are legion. Fortunately most people only get a mild dose, feel awful for a day or so and are more careful in future, but it takes an accident for them to learn. See the Garden Chemicals chapter and the Index, for more information.

Incorrect handling of dangerous chemicals

Once again these are often brought home from work, with less than a full appreciation of their toxicity. They can be strong acids, strong alkalis, or chemicals with pungent vapours and often they interact with each other or with moisture.

A friend told a young father of two to clean bricks with a mixture of pool chlorine, usually fairly safe, and hydrochloric acid. Unfortunately he mixed them inside his garage and was fatally overcome by the chlorine gas released by their interaction. Pool chlorine will also react with a small quantity of moisture to make an explosive mixture.

Petrol stored in large containers will occasionally explode if the vapour is ignited by a spark. Whenever there is a petrol strike reports of accidental swallowing of petrol while siphoning become more frequent. A few of these people end up in hospital with chemical pneumonia, others get petrol up their noses or Eustachian tubes where it burns the tender tissues.

Food poisoning

For a full discussion of this problem, see p. 7.

Allergic reactions

Allergic reactions are common and very hard to trace accurately. Once allergy to a chemical is suspected the only wise course of action is to avoid it. Quite often potent allergens carry warnings on their labels to the effect that contact with the skin may cause a rash, but most people don't read the fine print until after the rash has come up. It once took me three days to trace the reason for several fruit pickers' developing a severe rash. The fruit, it seemed, had been dusted with a chemical known to cause lumps in sensitive individuals. After doing a lot of research I spoke to the manufacturer, who told me that all the details were on the label, including the treatment!

FOOD POISONING

It is amazing how many people won't throw out a 20 cent can of beans unless they are absolutely sure it's dangerous. I would have thought the opposite more sensible — throw out everything unless you are sure of it. This is in fact the best advice for all canned goods. Despite carefully controlled manufacturing conditions, there are sometimes signs that the contents are a bit questionable — bulging can ends, spurting liquids, mould or a funny smell. Don't taste, just toss the food out.

Most people who ask my advice about using oldish food are too shy to say so, but seem to have a sneaking fear that a great disaster could occur if they use the food in question. The great disasters very rarely occur, but severe gastroenteritis can feel as though death is a preferable alternative.

Types of food poisoning

Botulism: This is the best-known and most feared of the food poisoning types. Australia has had only three reported cases of botulism. Two occurred when some canned beetroot escaped processing altogether and was thoroughly abnormal in appearance, taste and smell. The other case involved home preserved cantaloup (rockmelon). All occurrences involved underprocessing.

Vegetables, meat, some fruit, fish and poultry are nice and neutral and a suitable medium for growing the clostridium botulinum bacteria. It is wise not even to taste questionable foods because of the potency of the botulism toxin. To avoid botulism if you are a keen home preserver, keep to the instructions at all times.

Salmonella: This is present in lots of meats. It does not alter taste or smell and will reproduce very rapidly given warm, moist neutral conditions. Heat kills it but in poorly thawed poultry the centre of the bird may not reach a sufficiently high temperature during baking, so do thaw poultry well before cooking.

7

After cooking meats of all sorts, cool quickly and refrigerate as soon as possible — in this way you will keep bacterial counts of salmonella down.

Staphylococcal food poisoning: This is common in cold meats but also in egg-rich or milk-rich foods like custard, cream and mayonnaise. The source of the problem lies in a toxin produced by the bacteria. Heating will kill the bacteria but leaves the toxin intact. This type of food poisoning is once again common when food has been left in a warm spot for too long, but it does need initial careless food handling by people with pimples, boils and infected cuts or who are sneezing and coughing into food.

Vibrio parahaemolyticus: This type of food poisoning is almost exclusively associated with eating contaminated seafood and may develop up to 24 hours after ingestion. Everyone has heard of or been at a wedding where a dubious prawn cocktail has whipped the bride to her bed rather hurriedly.

Symptoms of food poisoning

Symptoms are usually abdominal colic or cramps, vomiting, diarrhoea and maybe a temperature. Salmonella may last for seven days but mostly, like the others, is over in 24 to 48 hours. If things become too uncomfortable, a doctor can relieve the extreme discomfort and prevent serious dehydration. Botulism differs from all other food poisonings in that people do die from it — in fact about 60 to 70 per cent of affected people die. The first symptoms of botulism aren't gastrointestinal, but are hoarseness, weakness, dizziness and headache. The patient becomes very ill rapidly once the symptoms begin, which is usually 12 to 36 hours after exposure.

Causes of food poisoning

Bacteria grow best in an environment which is warm, moist and neither acid nor alkaline. Very acid vegetables (tomatoes) and fruit (apples, peaches, citrus) are safe to preserve but most vegetables, meats and poultry need to be prepared with special apparatus at much higher temperatures to ensure safe eating. If you don't use high enough temperatures you are encouraging rapid reproduction of bacteria cells and in no time there is a certain case of food poisoning just waiting to happen.

Apart from preserved goods, food poisoning most often occurs when large quantities of food are prepared at one time, then left for four to five hours at a nice warm temperature. The explosive results may come on between two and 48 hours later and are due to contamination by one of a very small group of bacteria.

So here are some hints on how to avoid prostrating your family:

1. Don't keep food too long before using, especially if you prefer rare meat.

2. Keep your own standards of cleanliness up to scratch.

3. Store cooked food in the refrigerator immediately after serving. Your refrigerator won't heat to above 6°C if you put hot food in, and it's better to be quick.

4. Preserve all neutral foods under pressure for extended periods according to directions.

5. Thaw frozen foods completely before cooking or cook them for longer to compensate if you don't have the time.

6. You can safely re-freeze frozen foods if they are still cold to touch (i.e. about 40°F or 5°C) or have ice crystals on them and have been at this temperature no longer than two days. Generally, food that is safe to eat is safe to re-freeze. Anything that smells or looks odd, throw out.

GARDEN CHEMICALS

These days there aren't many very dangerous chemicals available for the home gardener — just a few. Lead arsenate, arsenic trioxide and phosphorus have all been replaced by chemicals less toxic to people but just as toxic to the aphids and red spider. This is no reason for complacency, however. Many of the newer chemicals need very careful handling. Parathion, for instance, is so toxic that to spill a few mls of the concentrated solution on to the skin would mean certain death. But then, no home gardener should use or need to use a chemical so strong.

There are literally thousands of chemicals used commercially. The most common are listed at the end of this chapter, with information on first symptoms, degree of danger, first aid, and precautions needed for safe use. Many chemicals used by gardeners can virtually be classed as non-toxic. It is a good idea to learn these, and regard all others as potentially dangerous, to be used carefully and only as their labels suggest.

Low toxicity garden chemicals

These include derris dust, pyrethrum, fertilisers, weedkillers except for paraquat and arsenic, antifungals, snail killers (toxic to dogs and poultry), white oil and sulphur. Of course, I am speaking in general terms — there are examples of poisonous chemicals in each group, but usually not in common usage. The best idea is to ring your local Poisons Information Centre or Department of Agriculture and ask about the specific chemicals you are using. I am also assuming that the above chemicals are being used correctly and not being taken in excess for the purposes of self-extinction — if you eat or drink enough of anything it will certainly make you sick.

Garden sprays

As I've said elsewhere, no one ever reads labels, and because of this garden sprays cause more accidental poisonings in adults than anything else.

Unlike nearly all other chemicals, the common garden sprays are absorbed through the skin very rapidly and completely. It is therefore essential not to spill or splash any on to clothes or bare skin, for this will have the same effect as taking a big swig out of the bottle. Because the label has been quickly scanned to find the dilution required and the rest of the blurb ignored, the innocent gardener leaves the splashes to dry. In half an hour he is beset by headache, nausea, streaming eyes and nose, funny tingling sensations and faintness and generally feels awful. Then he blames the spray.

Commonly, symptoms occur within an hour of misusing garden sprays. If the chemical is an organic phosphate they may consist of headache, dizziness, visual difficulty, nausea and salivation leading to more severe problems very rapidly when a large dose or a very toxic product is involved. Treatment is simply with atropine which is a rapid antidote. If the poisoning is too severe for atropine there is another drug, P.A.M., used these days which will be a sure cure — just so long as medical help is on the scene quickly enough. Speed is essential — and so is remembering to give the patient a good wash immediately, otherwise he will just keep absorbing more and more poison. In mild cases symptoms subside in three to four hours.

If the chemical is a chlorinated hydrocarbon the symptoms are also rapid in onset and begin with nausea but proceed to twitching, tremors and convulsions. Once again survival is dependent upon getting rapid medical aid. There is no specific antidote available for this group and treatment depends upon reducing symptoms as they arise and maintaining breathing and heart function.

Carbamates resemble organic phosphates in their toxicology and further than that I cannot go in general categories.

It is rare to become poisoned by breathing the fine spray of the insecticide, unless it is a very potent one, when a respirator and full protective gear should be worn. In normal garden usage the problems arise from spilled liquid concentrate and splashes on to clothes.

It is almost impossible to become poisoned by eating fruit or vegetables that have been recently sprayed because the sprays are very diluted in the form in which they are used and only a fine film is left. It is, however, wise to wash sprayed fruit and vegetables before eating, and to follow any instruction given on the insecticide label regarding the time which should be allowed between spraying and eating. I can remember one case where a lady helped herself to a large number of her neighbour's mulberries and got classical organic phosphate symptoms. She couldn't ask her neighbour what the mulberries had been sprayed with because she'd stolen them! After a couple of hours her nausea had gone.

People who have had a severe exposure to either of these two major groups of chemicals often complain that for several weeks or even months afterwards they don't feel themselves. They are often accused of malingering, but I don't believe that this is so. Somehow it takes a while for the body to sort itself out again, but once recovered there is no permanent damage.

Once a spray has been used outside, or inside by a pest controller (they use basically the same sorts of chemicals as described above), and the areas are dry, it is safe to let animals and children into the area. In the case of the persistent chemicals, i.e. the chlorinated hydrocarbons, much of the chemical evaporates as it dries, and with the organic phosphates the rate at which the chemical is destroyed in the atmosphere is rapid and the residue decreases speedily. The house will still smell awful, but don't be too worried — just open it up as much as possible for a few hours and then it will be safe to sleep in, despite a persistent odour that stays about for weeks. One thing to be careful of is puddles of spray — dogs and cats may drink them or walk through them, as may your child — so be sure to hose down the area where the mixing was done as a precaution.

Quite often I am asked about the safety of children playing in the garden while a neighbour is spraying for fruit fly, spiders, borers or anything else. It is very hard to be poisoned by inhalation out of doors (although it's certainly possible in confined spaces like under the house) so to be poisoned from yards away is impossible. Once again, however, it is just as well to keep children away from sprays, in case they become too interested and have their clothes or skin wet by them. If such an accident did occur a quick bath and change of clothing would prevent symptoms developing.

Weedkillers

Weedkillers are mostly of low toxicity but fairly irritant to the skin. A mouthful of 245T or chlorate will sting and cause vomiting but unless taken for suicidal purposes is unlikely to cause problems. The two exceptions are arsenic, of course, and paraquat. This latter chemical, particularly in its strong liquid form, a 20 per cent solution, leaves very few survivors even when only a mouthful has been accidentally swallowed. It is the same colour as cola and has often been put into a soft-drink bottle — then it's all over.

Fertilisers

Fertilisers are a bit irritating to the stomach — like having a drink of salt and water. None are really dangerous and a plate of icecream should fix things up, should they be ingested.

Safety precautions

1. Keep all chemicals out of the reach of your children or neighbour's children who may stray into your garage.

2. Label all your containers.

3. Read all the label carefully.

4. Wear protective clothing or at least long trousers, long-sleeved shirt, rubber gloves and boots.

5. Never prepare the diluted solutions in food containers or use them for storage.

6. Dispose of all residues after use.

7. Destroy superseded or unwanted stocks.

In summary — if you use chemicals properly they will be quite safe, no matter how potentially toxic they are. If you get a mild dose just sit it out; you'll know if you need a doctor or not because you are either mildly off-colour after the first hour or desperately ill. If you are seriously affected get to the nearest hospital post haste, waiting only to wash well and change your clothes.

Common agricultural chemicals

If the poisoning is serious call a doctor immediately—this first aid advice is only of help until medical assistance arrives.

Key

0 None   Harmful only under unusual conditions or in overwhelming dosage.
1 Slight   Causes mild symptoms which disappear at the end of the exposure.
2 Moderate   May cause strong symptoms but will not cause death or permanent injury.
3 High   May cause death or permanent injury but the amount required to do so depends upon the chemical. The asterisk* denotes a very high danger from a small quantity.

Chemical	Degree of danger (refer to key)	First symptoms of poisoning	First aid for swallowed poisons	Precautions for safe use
Organic Phosphates Demeton Dichlorvos Dimethoate Diazinon Fenthion Malathion (Maldison) Mevinphos Meta-systox *Parathion Rogor	Skin 3 Eye 3 Inhaled 3 Swallowed 3 Cumulative effect can occur in body.	Nausea, vomiting, abdominal pain, headaches, blurred vision. Apparent in 1 hour.	Induce vomiting immediately if swallowed. Wash all exposed skin, keep patient warm and quiet. Call doctor if exposure thought excessive.	Avoid skin contact, even with dry powder. Wear gloves, long sleeves and trousers (especially when using concentrate) and change any wet clothing. Avoid inhaling.

	Symptoms	Treatment	Notes
Carbamates Carbaryl Maneb Propoxur Thiram Zineb Ziram Skin 2 Eye 2 Swallowed 3 Inhaled 2 Cumulative effect can occur in body.	"	"	"
Chlorinated H/C *Aldrin Benzene hexa chloride (BHC) *Chlordane Chlordecone *Dieldrin D.D.T. *Endosulfan *Endrin *Heptachlor Lindane Methoxychlor Skin 3 Eye 3 Swallowed 3 Inhaled 3 Cumulative effect can occur in body.	Excitation, stimulation, twitches, difficulty with walking and if serious, convulsions. Apparent in $\frac{1}{2}$ hour.	"	"
Weedkillers *Paraquat and Diquat Skin 1 Eye 3 Swallowed 3 Inhaled 1 No cumulative effect in body.	Burns to mouth and tongue, vomiting, restlessness almost immediately.	Induce vomiting immediately and repeatedly, giving a drink of water between each vomit.	Not absorbed through skin very well, but care should be taken. **Never** make up solutions in food containers e.g. milk or soft drink bottles.
24D 245T TCA Chlorates Amitrole Atrazine MCPA MCPB Picloram Skin 1 Eye 2 Swallowed 1 Inhaled 1 No cumulative effect in body.	Nausea, vomiting and diarrhoea. May be delayed a couple of hours.	Induce vomiting if more than $\frac{1}{2}$ teaspoon eaten.	Not absorbed through skin but can irritate skin, so do not handle carelessly.

Chemical	Degree of danger (refer to key)	First symptoms of poisoning	First aid for swallowed poisons	Precautions for safe use
Dinoc DNOC	Skin 3 Eye 3 Swallowed 3 Inhaled 3 Cumulative effect can occur in body.	Nausea, vomiting, restlessness, sweating and flushed skin. Symptoms may be delayed several hours.	Induce vomiting immediately. Keep the patient cool as possible.	Particularly dangerous in hot weather and is absorbed through the skin. Wear gloves, shoes and long sleeves and trousers.
Rat and Rabbit Killers Warfarin	Skin 0 Eye 0 Swallowed 1 Inhaled 0 Cumulative effect can occur in body.	Bleeding occurs after eating some daily for several days.	For a single, small dose none is required.	Keep baits up high, away from children and animals.
*Phosphorus	Skin 3 Eye 3 Swallowed 3 Inhaled 3 Mild cumulative effect can occur in body.	Nausea, vomiting and diarrhoea in $\frac{1}{2}$ to 1 hour.	Induce vomiting immediately and repeatedly with a drink between vomits.	Keep baits up high, away from children and animals.
*Chloropicrin	Skin 3 Eye 3 Swallowed 3 Inhaled 3 Cumulative effect can occur in body.	Violent and immediate vomiting and diarrhoea. Tightness and pain in chest.	Give milk if possible. Keep patient warm till doctor arrives.	Never use without full body protection, plus protection against inhalation.
*1080	Skin 0 Eye 0 Swallowed 3 Inhaled 3 No cumulative effect in body.	Symptoms rarely begin before 2–3 hours, but are lethal if they do.	Immediate and repeated vomiting to wash stomach out. Drink water between each vomit.	Not absorbed through skin but otherwise use maximum protection.
*Cyanide	Skin 3 Eye 3 Swallowed 3 Inhaled 3 No cumulative effect in body.	Dizziness, rapid pulse and breathing and headache immediately.	If swallowed induce vomiting immediately and repeatedly with a drink between.	May be absorbed through skin, inhaled, or swallowed so use maximum protection.

	Ratings	Symptoms	Treatment	Precautions
Miscellaneous Bluestone (Copper Sulphate)	Skin 0 Eye 2 Swallowed 2 Inhaled 0 No cumulative effect in body.	Vomiting, burning pain in mouth and stomach immediately.	Induce vomiting and give milk and raw egg.	Do not use near children.
*Nicotine	Skin 3 Eye 3 Swallowed 3 Inhaled 3 No cumulative effect in body.	Violent vomiting, headache, blurred vision immediately.	Speed is essential. Give 8 teaspoonfuls of activated charcoal in water or if not available try to wash out stomach by repeated vomiting and drinking.	Wear protective clothing especially if using the concentrate. Store carefully.
Thiabendazole	Skin 0 Eye 1 Swallowed 1 Inhaled 0 No cumulative effect in body.	Dizziness, drowsiness and headache after an hour.	Induce vomiting.	Use carefully.
Carbon tetrachloride	Skin 3 Eye 3 Swallowed 3 Inhaled 3 Cumulative effect can occur in body.	Nausea, vomiting, dizziness, vagueness straight away.	Induce vomiting immediately and repeatedly.	*Never drink alcohol within 6–12 hours of using.* Caution at all times, especially for inhalation.
Mercurials	Skin 3 Eye 3 Swallowed 3 Inhaled 3 Cumulative effect can occur in body.	Vomiting, abdominal pain, bloody diarrhoea within an hour or so.	Induce vomiting.	General precautions. Avoid inhalation.
Pentachlorophenol	Skin 3 Eye 3 Swallowed 3 Inhaled 3 Cumulative effect can occur in body.	Fatigue, thirst, sweating, flushing of face, then vomiting, diarrhoea within an hour.	Induce vomiting. Give no fats or oils.	General precautions. Avoid inhalation.

POISONOUS PLANTS

I know of no case in which the death of a child was caused by eating a plant, but a great myth has built up around poisonous plants. It is very true that many plants are poisonous, but the important factor in determining toxicity is how much has been eaten. Stock frequently die through eating poisonous plants, but then they are herbivorous and eat nothing else — if you ate a whole celery patch you would develop a symptom or two, I'm sure. Quantity is the key word, and children just can't consume a whole tree of cassia beans. Because they don't, the symptoms which result from eating a leaf or two of *anything* are mostly non-existent or mild. The exceptions are marked in the following list of plants and it would be a good idea to remember only those with the triple asterisk. Stop worrying about your baby nibbling a bit of indoor plant or an odd frangipani leaf.

I once helped treat a galah that had eaten some mother-in-law's tongue and been rendered speechless and a kennel full of fox terriers that had eaten castor oil beans, but amongst humans genuine plant poisoning is extraordinarily rare. Castor oil beans are the most common serious offenders with children, and require immediate and intensive treatment.

There are seasonal trends depending upon what attractive berries are on the trees — winter for cotoneaster berries, autumn for ochna berries and cassia beans and summer for ornamental chilli. However, in almost all circumstances plant ingestions are harmless. Where poisonous plants have been eaten the quantity must be considered and if it seems dangerous **immediate** induction of vomiting (see First Aid chapter) is all that is required. If you can't identify the plant and you are going to worry, induce vomiting anyway; no harm will be done.

If the plant is burning the child's mouth, olive oil or butter rubbed around the cheeks and tongue followed by a big plate of icecream will settle the pain. Sometimes a burning mouth is accompanied by swollen lips, but the swelling should rapidly settle.

Children rarely eat more than a few leaves or berries of any plant because nature has protected them by making most poisonous plants vile tasting. If you suspect a poisoning try tasting the plant for yourself then smell or taste the saliva of your child. Where the taste is very strong and unpleasant common sense will mostly convince you that there can be nothing to worry about unless the offender is one of the half dozen dangerous plants.

Be on the lookout for your child's taking a fancy to a particular berry or seed. Children sometimes eat a few berries from an attractive shrub every day. These accumulate and may cause problems that one single dose would not. Even if the plant is harmless it is a good idea to dissuade them from the habit.

Adults rarely try eating strange plants, and adult poisoning by plants is rare. But I have had a few cases of accidental ingestion of hallucinogenic mushrooms (as opposed to the hundreds of cases of deliberate ingestion, see Drugs chapter) which to an unsuspecting person can be quite a surprising and unpleasant experience. One young couple were camping in a warm coastal area and cooked a large frypan full of mushrooms for breakfast in the years before the effects of hallucinogenic mushrooms were common knowledge. The husband managed to stop a passing car that took them to a doctor. The local doctor was quite baffled by the combination of their perfect physical health and wild mental state. The fantastic colour and music was appreciated by the husband who was an artist but his wife was still distressed by her bad "trip" weeks later.

LIST OF PLANTS

*May cause mild illness if large enough quantity eaten
**May cause symptoms but no danger to life
***Serious illness possible

Aconite (Monkshood): As for Delphinium.

African Violet: Not poisonous.

Agapanthus: Not poisonous.

Anemone: As for Delphinium.

***Angel's Trumpet** (*Datura arborea*): This is a small tree with soft hairy leaves. The trumpet-shaped flower is approximately 20 cm long and is white nerved with green. Induce vomiting immediately if more than half a leaf or a couple of seeds eaten. Symptoms begin within three hours and typically are dry throat, thirstiness, palpitations and flushed dry skin. Contact your local Poisons Information Centre or general practitioner.

*Apricot, Cherry, Plum, Peach kernels: If uncooked they contain small quantities of hydrocyanic acid. Ten to twenty kernels have caused symptoms in children. Induce vomiting if more than 10 have been eaten, otherwise no treatment is necessary.

Ardisia: Not poisonous.

**Arum Lily: All parts of these common white lilies will cause a burning pain in the mouth if eaten, due to the presence of quite high concentrations of oxalic acid. Children typically come running for help, crying and screaming, due to the intense pain and for this reason only small quantities are ever eaten and there is no chance of serious illness.

Give milk and icecream to cool the burning pain. The calcium in these foods will inactivate the oxalate causing the trouble. Skin dermatitis has also been reported.

Asparagus Fern berries: Not poisonous.

Aspidistra: Not poisonous.

Atropa belladonna: See Deadly Nightshade.

Azalea: The leaves and stems contain a cardiac glycoside but poisoning will occur only after eating a large quantity.

Begonia: Not poisonous.

*Belladonna Lily: As for Arum Lily.

Bird of Paradise: (Strelitzia): Not poisonous.

Brunfelsia: Not poisonous.

Buddleia: Not poisonous.

*Bulbs: Bulbs of any plant should not be eaten, but generally they taste so awful that only one or two bites could possibly be swallowed. If you suspect that a lot has been eaten, induce vomiting immediately, observe the child for two hours and call your local Poisons Information Centre or GP if worried.

*Buttercup: May cause skin irritation or dermatitis and when eaten causes a burning sensation in the mouth. This would irritate the stomach and intestines too, causing both vomiting and diarrhoea, but these symptoms have only ever been observed in stock. Give large quantities of milk to dilute the poison.

Cactus Plants: Not poisonous

Calendula: See Marigold.

Camellia: Not poisonous.

*Candelabra Cactus: See Poinsettia.

Cape Lilac: See White Cedar.

*Capsicum: See Chilli.

*Cassia: This is a very commonly eaten plant and is not poisonous although eating very large numbers of pods or eating a few pods daily for a week or so have caused diarrhoea and vomiting.

***Castor Oil beans: A very common plant on waste land, the Castor Oil plant grows up to four and a half metres high with large leaves, greenish-white to rust coloured flowers and spiny seed capsules containing three seeds. It is only chewed seeds that are dangerous but two to three of these are sufficient to cause serious illness.

Symptoms may be delayed up to 36 hours after ingestion but more commonly begin after a couple of hours. The most obvious symptom is bloody diarrhoea. If the child is even suspected of eating any beans, vomiting must be induced immediately and the child taken straight to hospital.

Celery: Not poisonous but vast quantities of green leaves have caused gastritis in cows.

*Cherry kernels: See Apricot kernels.

*Chilli: The offending plant is most commonly the attractive ornamental chilli whose fruits cause immediate severe burning pain in the mouth. Rub the child's mouth with olive oil or butter and give plenty of icecream or cold milk and soon all symptoms will have gone.

*Christmas Rose (Hellebore): Same as for Buttercup.

Chrysanthemum: Not poisonous but causes a mild stinging sensation in the mouth. It has also caused dermatitis in sensitive people. Give cold milk to stop the burning.

*Clivia (Kaffir Lily): Same mild problems as for Daffodil.

**Colocasia (Taro): As for Arum Lily.

Convolvulus (Morning Glory): The seeds of one U.S. species contain an hallucinogenic ingredient but the common garden morning glory is not this species. Not poisonous.

Cornflower: Not poisonous.

Cotoneaster: Not poisonous but eating the berries should be discouraged.

Crataegus: Berries are frequently eaten but are not poisonous.

*Crown of Thorns: See Poinsettia.

**Cunjevoi: As for Arum Lily.

Cyclamen: The tuber is poisonous but because it has an acrid, bitter taste, poisoning is rare. If more than half a tuber has been eaten, medical attention is advised.

*Daffodil: Both the stems and bulbs contain active principles likely to cause vomiting and diarrhoea, but unless the equivalent of one plant is eaten, symptoms are unlikely. When mistaken for onions has caused gastritis.

Dahlia: Not poisonous.

Daisy: All varieties may cause the same mild problems as chrysanthemums. See Chrysanthemum.

Dandelion: Not poisonous.

**Daphne: All parts are poisonous, especially the berries, but children rarely eat this plant. It causes severe gastroenteritis with vomiting and diarrhoea beginning after a couple of hours. Skin allergies occur occasionally too. If more than one to two leaves or berries are eaten, induce vomiting immediately and give large quantities of milk. Contact your local Poisons Information Centre or doctor if worried.

***Deadly Nightshade (*Atropa belladonna*): A perennial about 1 metre high with pointed oval leaves about 15 cm long. The single flowers emerging from the joint of the leaf and stem are blue-purple or dull red bells about 2·54 cm long. The berry is round, about 1·27 cm wide and is purple to shiny black when ripe.

Poisoning is extremely rare even in countries where the plant grows wild, but if you have this plant growing, it would be wise to pull it out. For symptoms and treatment see Angel's Trumpet.

*Delphinium: This species of plant has been shown to be a problem with cattle and sheep who like eating it in large quantities, but human poisoning has never been reported. The amount likely to be eaten casually by a child would cause no harm — at worst some mild diarrhoea. Give milk and food to dilute. Sensitive skin may show allergy to these plants.

**Dieffenbachia: As for Arum Lily.

**Dumb Cane (Dieffenbachia): As for Arum Lily.

Elder: The berries may cause nausea if uncooked but once cooked are no problem.

**Elephant's Ears: As for Arum Lily.

Forget-me-not: Not poisonous.

***Foxglove: Although this common garden plant is the source of the much used drug, digitalis, reports of poisoning of children are very rare. One case reported was a mild intoxication which resulted from a two-year-old's drinking the water from a vase which had contained these flowers. The only other case on record reports a child chewing many seeds. If you have this plant in your garden and your child does eat everything he touches, it may be wise to take it out just for a year or two till he grows out of this habit. If you discover or suspect that any has been eaten, induce vomiting immediately and observe closely for three to six hours for vomiting, diarrhoea, abdominal pain, headache or any distinct change in condition. Go straight to hospital if any of these symptoms appear.

Frangipani: Not poisonous, but give milk to get rid of the objectionable taste.

Freesia: Not poisonous, but the bulbs may cause mild stinging in the mouth if they are chewed. Give milk to wash the mouth clean.

Fuchsia: Not poisonous.

Gardenia: Not poisonous.

Geranium: Not poisonous, but may cause skin allergy in sensitive people.

Gladioli: Not poisonous, but may cause a burning sensation in the mouth. Give milk to wash mouth clean.

Gloxinia: Not poisonous.

Gum Trees: Not poisonous in quantities likely to be eaten by children, but a couple of species have caused problems with cattle in times of drought. Give milk.

Hawthorn (Crataegus): The bright orange berries attract children but are not poisonous.

*Hellebore: See Christmas Rose.

Hibiscus: Not poisonous.

*Holly: Said to cause vomiting and diarrhoea if more than 20 berries eaten but the prickles on the leaf make it unlikely that this would occur. If worried induce vomiting immediately.

*Hyacinth: Ten bulbs eaten by a two-year-old may cause violent diarrhoea. Skin allergy from just touching the plant has also been reported. If bulbs are eaten, induce vomiting to prevent purging.

Hydrangea: Mild gastroenteritis and nausea occurred in one family when the children added hydrangea buds to a tossed salad, but under normal circumstances the symptoms would not seem severe enough to warrant treatment other than a drink of milk.

Iris: The bulb is extremely unpalatable and unlikely to be eaten, but like the rest of the plant may cause mild gastroenteritis. Serious poisoning is unknown. Give milk to minimise irritation. Skin irritations after handling the plant have been reported.

*Ivy: A few cases of mild poisoning in children when "very considerable" numbers of the berries were reported to have caused diarrhoea. If only a couple of berries eaten just give milk, but for 10 to 20 berries, induce vomiting immediately. Dermatitis resulting from handling the plant has been reported.

Jacaranda: Not poisonous.

Jade Plant: Not poisonous.

*****Jonquil:**   See Daffodil.

Kaffir Lily: See Clivia.

******Laburnum:**   This is not a common tree in Australia but there are many English reports of children eating one to two pods. All vomited within minutes and other observed symptoms include drowsiness, weakness and palpitation.

Give large quantities of milk and contact your local Poisons Information Centre or medical practitioner.

*********Lantana:**   There are several reports of quite serious poisoning in children as a result of eating green lantana berries. Symptoms, beginning two to six hours after ingestion, include weakness, vomiting, dilated pupils and slow deep breathing.

It is most important to induce vomiting immediately, then no symptoms will develop. Immediately upon discovery of the ingestion take the child to hospital.

*****Larkspur:**   See Delphinium.

Lilac: Not poisonous.

Lilli Pilli: Not poisonous.

*****Lilies:**   There are a vast number of varieties. A few are poisonous but most only cause a local sting in the mouth and, if sufficient has been eaten, diarrhoea and vomiting. A glass of cold milk or some icecream is usually the best treatment. Check under the specific name of the lily.

******Lily of the Valley:**   Supposed to be poisonous, but there have been no specific cases reported. To play safe, if your child eats a couple of leaves or a stem of flowers induce vomiting immediately and observe carefully for the next 24 hours for vomiting, diarrhoea, weakness and headache

******Lobelia:**   All parts of this plant are poisonous, but severe symptoms in children have not been reported. Should much of it be eaten, vomiting will occur within half an hour followed by sweating and a rapid pulse. It would be a wise precaution to induce vomiting immediately the ingestion occurs to avoid symptoms developing, if possible.

*****Lupin:**   There is massive evidence of stock poisoning but no human ingestions have been reported. The new green shoots and the pods and their seeds are the most poisonous parts so if your child eats much immediate induction of vomiting would be a good idea.

Marigold: Not poisonous but may cause a stinging sensation in mouth. Give milk to wash it off the tongue and cheeks and to dilute it.

*Monkshood: As for Delphinium.

Monstera: The leaves may cause a mild burning sensation in the mouth if they are chewed. Rinse the mouth well and give cold milk to ease the stinging.

Moreton Bay Fig: Not poisonous.

Morning Glory: See Convolvulus.

**Mother-in-Law Plant: See Arum Lily.

Nasturtium: Not poisonous.

Oak: Acorns and leaves are poisonous to stock, but it would be impossible for children to eat them in quantities large enough to cause a problem.

Ochna: The berries are frequently eaten by children but are not poisonous.

***Oleander: Although this is a very common garden shrub poisonings by it are extremely rare. Human deaths have been reported, but such cases are poorly described. The taste of the sap is very bitter indeed and it is almost impossible to imagine a child persevering long enough to eat a lethal amount. Symptoms would begin with vomiting and diarrhoea.

If your child has eaten any part of the tree, immediately induce vomiting just to be safe and observe for six hours for vomiting or any change in condition. Contact your local Poisons Information Centre or doctor.

Skin allergies to oleander are common.

Orchids: Not poisonous.

*Ornamental Chilli: See Chilli.

Pansy: Not poisonous.

Peach: See Apricot.

*Pencil Tree: See Poinsettia.

*Pepper Tree: The fruit is irritant when eaten and may cause a burning sensation in the mouth and mild gastroenteritis. Wash mouth out well and give cold milk to drink.

*Philodendron: Some species may cause a mild stinging in the mouth. Rub olive oil or butter in the mouth and give cold milk or icecream. Loose bowel motions may be observed, but this should be short lived. Skin allergies have been occasionally reported.

Pigface: Not poisonous, in the quantity likely to be eaten by children.

Plum: See Apricot.

*Poinsettia and other Euphorbias (Crown of Thorns, Snow on the Mountain, Pencil Tree, Candelabra Cactus):   The milky sap from all of these plants will cause blistering on the skin and so if sucked by a child will cause an immediate stinging pain in the mouth. This also makes ingestion of more than one mouthful extremely unlikely.

Dilution of the acrid principle with milk and food and oils should be sufficient to stop the symptoms and prevent diarrhoea and vomiting occurring.

If the sap gets into the eyes immediately flood for five minutes with warm water. If the eye remains sore and swollen for more than 12 hours see a doctor.

**Poison Ivy: See Rhus.

Poppy: Not poisonous.

Potato: The vines, sprouts and sun-spoiled green potatoes have caused stock poisoning, but so long as all the green is pared from the potato and it is cooked there is no danger of poisoning.

Primrose: Not poisonous, but has caused dermatitis in sensitive people.

Privet: The berries in very large numbers would probably cause vomiting and diarrhoea, but cases of poisoning in children are virtually unknown. A drink of milk and some food should be adequate to prevent irritation of the stomach.

Prunus: See Apricot.

Rhododendron: See Azalea.

**Rhubarb: The leaf (not the leaf stalk) contains large amounts of oxalic acid and is therefore potentially dangerous and should not be eaten raw or cooked. Several whole leaves would need to be eaten before the poisoning became severe. Symptoms of excessive salivation, vomiting and diarrhoea would be expected after one to two hours.

Give large quantities of milk as this will inactivate the oxalic acid before any damage can be done. If a large quantity has been eaten, immediate induction of vomiting is essential.

**Rhus: Dermatitis may be caused by touching broken parts of the plant or handling animals, clothing or implements which have touched broken stems. There is no evidence that unbroken stems or leaves give off any poisonous exudate. The plant is toxic all year round. The dermatitis is manifested by reddened and itchy skin in mild cases and blisters which exude serum in severe cases, when infection is a real danger.

Eating of the leaves or fruit by a sensitive person is very dangerous; the dermatitis-like reaction also takes place in the mouth, stomach and intestines causing serious gastric upset. About half the population is estimated to be sensitive to the plant, and those who are not sensitive do not develop any symptoms whatever. It is not possible to get a reaction without actually touching the plant or a carrier (shoes, clothing, garden tools, pets).

Should contact occur wash the area immediately. This will not prevent the reaction occurring, just prevent transmission. Seek medical advice if blisters develop.

The smoke from burning Rhus is also allergenic.

Rose: Not poisonous.

Rubber Tree Plant: Not poisonous.

Saxifrage: As for Hydrangea.

*Snow on the Mountain: See Poinsettia.

Strawberries, wild: Not poisonous.

Strelitzia: Not poisonous.

Sweet-Pea: Continuous eating of the seeds has caused poisoning in stock, but this has not been reported with children. All the same, do not allow your child to get a taste for the seeds, just in case.

**Taro: See Arum Lily.

**Toadstools: No one has died from eating these in Australia but there are a few varieties which cause symptoms. Symptoms begin within a couple of hours and may be severe vomiting and diarrhoea, or hilarity or hallucinations. They are easily controlled in hospital. The toadstool species which cause adverse effects rarely look like the edible mushrooms. The round puff-balls that spring up in abundance after rain are non-poisonous, as are the small spindly pale-coloured toadstools that accompany them in everyone's backyard after a good storm.

If you have picked what you think are field mushrooms and you're in doubt, don't use them — they could be one of the non-edible varieties. There is no easy way to distinguish the safe from the unsafe.

*Tomato: The leaves of the tomato taste most unpleasant and ingestion is therefore unlikely. If quite a large quantity is eaten, gastritis should be expected.

Violet: Not poisonous.

Violet, African: Not poisonous.

Virginia Creeper: There is some suspicion, but no evidence, that the berries may be poisonous, causing vomiting and diarrhoea. If many (say, 10) have been eaten, induce vomiting immediately just to be on the safe side.

Wandering Jew: Not poisonous, but causes skin allergies in some people.

Wattle: Not poisonous in quantities likely to be taken by children.

**White Cedar or Cape Lilac: Fruits have caused severe dehydration because of vomiting and diarrhoea but these symptoms can be controlled in hospital. The berries have a foul odour and taste, so poisonings are rare.

Wistaria: Not poisonous.

*Yew: Very rarely eaten, but a large quantity of the leaves and seeds will cause gastritis.

DRUGS

Drugs may be defined as chemical substances which affect the body or mind, or both. Thus, this chapter is concerned not only with those substances usually meant when "the drug problem" is discussed — marihuana, cocaine, L.S.D. and the rest — but also painkillers, alcohol, tranquillisers, nicotine and other commonplace drugs used and abused by large numbers of people.

Many drugs can be and are of great benefit to society, relieving pain, conquering disease, helping people under stress, and so on, when they are used intelligently and responsibly. But unfortunately the drugs can be most harmful when used to excess, for the wrong reasons, or at the wrong times. When abused in this way either intentionally or by accident, the most helpful drug can become a "poison".

I will discuss the misuse of drugs under four headings: Domestic Drug Abuse, Recreational Drug Abuse, Deliberate Sedative Overdose, and Effects of Drugs on the Foetus and Breastfed Baby.

DOMESTIC DRUG ABUSE

At some time it is necessary for everyone to have a tablet of the kind that fits into the category of home abused drugs. I class painkillers, alcohol, nicotine, diet pills, caffeine, tranquillisers and a few other rare things in this group.

To use a drug is to take it when necessary to relieve the condition for which it is prescribed. To abuse a drug is to take it for any other reason. Remember there is a great difference.

Painkillers

Analgesics are very useful for babies' teething problems, headaches, muscular aches and pains and a variety of other things so well described on the packet. Read the rest of the packet and you will find the suggested dosages which should be adhered to. Some people might think it unbelievable that quite a sizeable proportion of the population take one or two packets of analgesics every day. Man's insatiable desire to take medicine is the basis of the psychology of this extraordinary syndrome.

The abuser thinks that he may get a headache, so takes a powder on rising in the morning just in case a headache should develop. The caffeine present in the powder helps to give him a lift and start the day well. Psychologically he has now taken a magic substance that will keep him going till lunchtime (or perhaps only till morning tea). At the slightest emotional upset (and don't we all have plenty of those) — another powder.

Five to 10 years of this abuse, and the kidneys are gradually affected and damaged. As time goes by more and more of the kidneys are destroyed. It is still not known for certain which ingredient or combination of ingredients is responsible, but so long as you use and don't abuse these useful tablets your kidneys will be fine. Next time you reach for the bottle think twice — is your head really so bad that in 10 minutes it won't be better? Your hangover will be there whether you take a painkiller or not — everyone knows there is no cure for that disease.

Alcohol

It would be impossible to assess the misery and distress caused by alcohol. It is very pleasant to use alcohol to relax and let yourself unwind, whether at a party or at home. It is useful as a nightcap, it is an excellent sedative, but these are USES.

Unhealthy drinking habits are usually obvious by about the age of 30. It is a habit to feel that you need four drinks (or eight or 10) before dinner, or half a dozen schooners every night at the hotel before coming home to face the family chaos. To prevent these habits developing often requires a lot of self-control — it is so easy to anaesthetise yourself into a groggy state and let the world pass by without upsetting you.

As the years pass and the habit gets worse, so the number of destroyed brain cells increases and a different personality develops. Days are lost from work, jobs are not held long, money needed for other things is wasted on alcohol. Life with the alcoholic is intolerable even for the saints and martyrs of this world. The cost to the community of the loss to the workforce, the support of the neglected family and the hospital bills due to alcohol-related diseases is enormous.

The answer is not prohibition — it is **use** of alcohol, as opposed to **abuse**. Successful recovery from the disease of alcoholism is rare — almost all alcoholics die alcoholics.

Nicotine

Similarly, few cigarette smokers successfully conquer their addiction (or dependence, which is the more correct term to use).

Unfortunately, like the other addictions discussed, smoking is a health hazard, and after years of heavy smoking all sorts of fatal diseases tend to develop. I don't think it is possible to **use** cigarettes — use and abuse are here indistinguishable. One recent paper claimed that even one to five cigarettes daily significantly shorten life expectancy, so it is quite staggering to assess the years of life lost because of heavy smoking.

Once again it is also the community's burden; before the final demise there are the inevitable spells in hospital chest wards — years, perhaps, of emphysema preventing useful or pleasurable living. So it is better not to start — but who cares about being 65 when you are only 15? Almost nobody.

Diet pills

Diet pills are no longer a big problem. The stimulants that were used as the major ingredient of such pills have been almost phased out, and occur only in a few pills which are available on medical prescription.

The problem began because the happy-go-lucky feeling the pills gave tended to replace dieting as the reason for taking them. If you wake up feeling really glum and sad how marvellous to take a pill and, presto, feel on top of the world. No wonder they were a success. Why, you may ask, should people not be allowed this easy way to happiness? Once again, nothing is so easy. After a few hours the stimulation decreased and was replaced by mild depression, so obviously at that stage many people took another tablet. And after taking these tablets for a few months or years, larger doses were needed to achieve the same happiness and the depression, a few hours later, was no longer mild. More tablets, more depression and so the vicious cycle developed, as a result of **abuse** replacing **use**. Some people who built up to huge daily doses also suffered personality changes and severe mental disturbance, even after the tablets were discontinued.

Today in Australia this situation is very rare and diet medications are safe.

Caffeine

One bright spot in this chapter is that caffeine will give most people a bit of a lift if they are feeling droopy, but has no long term sinister effects (if we disregard a recent proposal that excesses of caffeine are involved in the development of heart disease). Just so long as you don't mind the diuretic effect that accompanies the mild stimulation (an excessive amount of urine is made), you can drink coffee, tea, cola and cocoa to your heart's content. All of these drinks contain caffeine, but it is very difficult to abuse them, unless you are suffering from heart damage. Large amounts of caffeine can cause sleeplessness.

Tranquillisers

I will give you my opinions here; they differ from those of other people but there is no way I could cover the sociological, medical and psychological sides of the argument.

I think that living happily is difficult for everyone but nobody has anything like the answer to society's unhappiness and failure to cope. Overdoses are so common they are no longer worthy of a raised eyebrow, crime is an outlet for some, alternative societies are being established with varying success by others.

For all of us life must continue. Some people are helped in the short term by tranquillisers. Used sensibly, and according to medical advice, tranquillisers cut out a lot of unnecessary worrying and enable the business of living to go on. It surely can't be better to suffer, so a blanket ruling out of all sedatives is quite uncharitable and senseless. Because there is evidence that tranquillisers can cause acute anxiety if they are stopped abruptly after continuous treatment, producing real "withdrawal symptoms", it is best to have a healthy respect for them, but I do say: Go ahead, have a tablet **if you need it**. There are, of course, those who vastly exceed the recommended doses — but in these cases the doctor has probably not recognised the depth of the problem and could have prescribed something more suitable with added help from a social worker, psychoanalyst or community self-help centre. Such centres are places where discussion and interaction with others make it quite obvious that the patient isn't the only sad person about. Somehow there is strength in community feeling. Sitting at home and watching TV all day every day apart from the few hours spent doing essential work is the ideal formula for a boredom-based neurotic disease. Get out and get going — and you'll survive our crazy rat race so much more sanely. And above all, stop enjoying being sick!

RECREATIONAL DRUG ABUSE

The psychology of the dependent drug user is too complex for me to discuss here. The basic reason for drug-taking seems to be the desire to escape the realities of life. The users just can't cope, and it's nice to get away for a while into another, more pleasant, world.

Serious drug abuse is the result of the interaction of many factors, including the psychological state of the person, his friends, his home, his personality. It is hard to pick any particular personality type more likely than another to become dependent on drugs.

The experimental use of drugs is quite different. Drugs must be fun and must be pleasant or the current situation would never have developed. Most experimenters with marihuana never progress to other drugs, in the same way that most people who enjoy a drink before dinner don't progress to methylated spirits in the gutter.

For the parent with teenagers it is important to have trust in your child and play the whole question of drugs down. Don't fly off the handle, don't be forever asking leading questions, don't search his room. Try to discuss the question openly. If you do discover some marihuana (pot, grass) or he admits having smoked some, don't think that it is the end — just take a deep breath and try to be un-impressed (it was probably said to shock you). Then open up a conversation on a friendly level.

If all this sounds too difficult for your case, above all don't throw the child out of the house in rage but leave it and try to find out more facts from people who provide advice on these matters, for example the Health Commission's Mental Health and Drug Education Section, a Drug Referral Centre, or one of the other many places that exist in all large cities to provide such help.

"Drugs" frighten parents because they do not understand the actions, good or bad, that each abused drug can bring on, and they do not understand why anyone would want to have a "high". Have you ever wondered why you like that drink after work, or those many drinks at a party?

The following table is reprinted from the pamphlet *Drugs: A Social Issue*, published by the Health Commission of New South Wales:

34 *Is it Poisonous?*

Drug Group	Name	Origin	Medical Use	How Taken	Psych. Dep.*
	Heroin	Opium poppy	None in Australia	Sniffed /Injected	Yes
	Morphine	Opium poppy	Painkiller	Injected	Yes
NARCOTICS	Codeine	Opium poppy	For cough	Swallowed	Yes
	Pethidine	Synthetic	Painkiller	Swallowed /Injected	Yes
	Methadone	Synthetic	Withdrawal from heroin	Swallowed /Injected	Yes
	Barbiturates	Synthetic	Sleep and sedation	Swallowed /Injected	Yes
	Alcohol	Grain & fruit	Limited	Swallowed	Yes
SEDATIVES	Minor Tranquillisers	Synthetic	Tension and anxiety	Swallowed	Yes
	Inhalants & Solvents i.e. Glues & Aerosol sprays	Synthetic	Mostly none	Inhaled	Yes
	Nicotine	Tobacco leaves	None	Inhaled	Yes
	Amphetamine	Synthetic	Strictly limited medical use in Australia	Swallowed /Injected	Yes
STIMULANTS	Cocaine	Coca leaves	Local anaesthetic	Sniffed /Injected	Yes
	Caffeine	Coffee bean Kola nut Synthetic Tea leaves	Mild stimulant	Swallowed	Yes
ANALGESICS	Aspirin & many other Tablets & Powders	Synthetic	Painkiller	Swallowed	Yes

*Psychological Dependence

Phys. Dep.**	Short Term Effects	Long Term Effects
Yes		
Yes	Last approx. 2 hours. Relief of pain and anxiety, feelings of well-being, decreased awareness of outside world. Vomiting, drowsiness and sleep in some individuals. High doses can cause unconsciousness and death.	Physical and psychological dependence. Withdrawal symptoms—tremors, vomiting, insomnia, pain and weight loss. Self-injection with dirty syringe can cause hepatitis, abscesses and septicaemia (blood poisoning). Risk of death by overdose is very high.
Yes		
Yes		
Yes		
Yes	Last 4–8 hours. Relaxation, happy feeling, drowsiness, lack of attention, and sleep. Large dose can cause death.	Convulsions when withdrawing are severe enough to cause death. Overdose is the cause of many accidental deaths and suicides.
Yes	Last 2–4 hours. Relaxation, feelings of happiness and well-being. Large doses may cause unconsciousness and hangover.	Continued heavy use may result in alcoholism, brain, heart and liver damage and sometimes death.
Yes	Last 12–24 hours. Relief of anxiety and tension. Large doses may cause drowsiness, blurred vision and sleep.	Continued heavy use may destroy blood cells and bring on coma.
No	Last 1–3 hours. Feelings of happiness, relaxation and drowsiness. Large amounts may cause illness and death by suffocation.	Liver, kidney and brain damage may result.
Yes	Last ¼–2 hours. Relaxation, headache, loss of appetite and nausea.	Heart and lung disease, cancer, bronchitis and breathing difficulties.
No	Last 4–8 hours. Highly stimulating. Causes excited state, increased activity and decreased appetite. Large doses may cause inability to sleep.	Inability to sleep, high degree of excitation, skin complaints, malnutrition and mental illness.
No	Last 4 hours. Cause feeling of self-confidence and power, decreased fatigue and loss of hunger.	Damage to mucous membranes around nose. Sleeplessness and mental illness.
No	Last 2–4 hours. Cause increased alertness. Large doses may cause inability to sleep.	Restlessness. Caffeine is harmful to people with heart damage.
No	Last 1–4 hours. Relief of pain. If preparation contains caffeine, it may cause stimulant effect.	Continued heavy use can result in kidney disease, stomach bleeding and anaemia.

**Physical Dependence

Drug Group	Name	Origin	Medical Use	How Taken	Psych. Dep.*
HALLUCINOGENS	S.T.P. L.S.D. D.M.T. **Mescaline** **Psilocybin**	Synthetic Synthetic Synthetic Cactus Psilocybe mushroom	L.S.D. has been tested for treat- ment of psychiatric illness but is no longer being used for this. No other med- ical uses of these drugs.	Swallowed Swallowed Swallowed Swallowed Swallowed	Yes Yes Yes Yes Yes
HALLUCINOGEN- INTOXICANT	**Marihuana**	Cannabis plant	No present med. use.	Swallowed /Inhaled	Yes

*Psychological Dependence

DELIBERATE OVERDOSE

Attempted suicides are increasing at an alarming rate and occurring in younger and younger age groups. In my experience of those cases where suicide has obviously not been the aim, the patient is making a grand gesture to the world or someone in particular saying "I can't cope." Very often hospital treatment of the overdose is not necessary in these cases, and is vigorously fought by the patient, who just needs tender loving care from someone who hasn't been giving it.

Consider the question of deliberately ingested overdose. There are many problems in such cases, often the patient refuses all treatment and it is not known if the number of tablets claimed to have been taken has in fact been taken. Try very hard to ascertain what was swallowed, the strength of the tablet, the number originally in the bottle, and get an exact history of when they were swallowed. If, after receiving medical advice about the overdose, there is no immediate medical problem, do not neglect the need for future psychological help. If the gesture involved just a few aspirin or something you are sure is safe, psychological help is all that is required.

Phys. Dep.**	Short Term Effects	Long Term Effects
No No No No No	Last 6–12 hours. Cause hallucinations, i.e. the user sees lights, colours, designs and feels very aware of things happening inside and outside the body. Anxious feelings and panic due to loss of control may be experienced.	Chromosome damage has been reported but is unproven. May cause attempted suicide, depression, "flashback" experience and in some people mental illness.
No	Last 2–4 hours. Relaxation, laughter, increased appetite, slowing down of time. Dry mouth, dizziness, blood shot eyes and decreased co-ordination may occur. A panic reaction may occur in some users.	High tar intake of heavy users may cause respiratory complications. The active ingredient (THC) is stored in the body. It is not known whether it may become active at some later stage. Heavy use by those with personality difficulties can cause problems.

**Physical Dependence

If you can see that it has been an overdose of some magnitude, with increasing drowsiness progressing to deep sleep then hospital is essential. It is often difficult to tell the difference between unconsciousness and deep sleep and there are too many hazards involved in being in this state at home — vomiting while asleep and inhaling the vomit into the lung is quite common, and may cause death or at least pneumonia. Don't think that just because the patient is sleeping peacefully it is safe to leave him — it isn't.

In hospital the treatment of sleeping tablet overdose is very simple and relies on keeping up the blood pressure, keeping up the breathing, and preventing or treating complications like vomiting or decreases in breathing which may, if untreated, lead to brain damage from lack of oxygen. If these things are done then nature does the rest and finally, depending on the dose taken, the patient wakes up, feeling very groggy and depressed.

Cases of attempted suicide are not reported to the police and I truly believe that they have no role whatever to play in the matter — it is a purely medical problem.

If you find yourself involved in a case of attempted suicide make sure you collect all the information you can about what was taken, how, where and when. Also, before taking on the responsibility of leaving the patient at home, check with a doctor. After the episode is over the most important part of all is making sure that everything possible is done to straighten out the reason for the attempt in the first place. A friendly local G.P., a minister or priest, a trusted parent, a psychiatrist — someone must intervene to help sort out the psychological problems which led to the patient's taking this serious step.

For first aid while getting to hospital see pp. 60-61.

EFFECTS OF DRUGS ON THE FOETUS AND BREASTFED BABY

Effects of drugs on the foetus

Drugs were known to be capable of killing or malforming embryos long before thalidomide was discovered, and some much-used chemicals are only just coming under suspicion. No one really knows for sure why a baby can be affected and his mother left unscathed, but while they are finding out I would think it only sensible to avoid *all* sources of foreign chemicals for the first 12 to 15 weeks of pregnancy. That means avoiding exposure to garden sprays, vapours, dusts and fumes at work, and even the chemicals present in ready-prepared foods. Remember, too, that rubella (German measles) vaccination, smallpox vaccination and X-rays can cause foetal damage and must be avoided. At the other end of pregnancy it is important that nothing affects the ability of the baby to survive labour and the immediate postnatal period, so drugs should be kept to a minimum then too.

Chemicals and drugs by themselves cannot cause a malformed foetus. There are always other factors involved, such as genetic background, maternal age and the susceptibility of the foetus at that particular time. The birth of a deformed baby is therefore never a foregone conclusion because of a single event. Even mothers who catch rubella (German measles) in the first few weeks of pregnancy don't always give birth to an affected baby — it's just that the odds are extremely high. Fortunately there are more and more tests becoming available to demonstrate the viability and normality of the baby within the first 12 to 15 weeks of pregnancy.

In its first 15 weeks of life, factors from the environment can affect the embryo dramatically, causing physical defects such as congenital heart malformation, spina bifida, cleft palate, absent limbs, hearing and visual defects. It is during this crucial 15-week period that all the basic work in forming organs is done.

In the period 15 to 40 weeks there are a few commonly used and readily available drugs that cause problems, but by far the worst is tobacco. Even five cigarettes per day can result in a reduced birth weight, so imagine the effect of 40 per day! It is becoming clear as a result of recent research that alcohol, and aspirin and other pain-killing preparations, taken excessively or daily, and hard drugs, are causing a higher incidence of abnormal babies. It is important to avoid constant high-level exposure to any of these during pregnancy. During the 15- to 40-week period, also, some hormones intended to affect only the mother can affect the baby, for example antithyroid drugs can give the baby a goitre and oestrogens may feminise a male foetus. These are usually fairly mild and transient problems, but it would be better if they didn't occur at all.

So as a general rule avoid everything except the very natural for the first 15 weeks. Don't smoke, avoid large doses and varieties of drugs for the rest of the pregnancy, and try hard not to contract any diseases especially rubella. Although flu, chicken pox and some less common infections have been recently subjected to scrutiny the results were inconclusive. That means that the disease may influence the development of a foetus in one case in a thousand or it may, on the other hand, have no effect in any of them.

Any drugs that are definitely known to affect the embryo and cause major structural deformities are not on the market (except for a few special drugs for cancer) and those that affect the baby in the 15- to 40-week period are not prescribed for pregnant women or used only when absolutely essential, bearing in mind that the risk to the foetus is either small or transient in nature. Always be sure that your doctor knows you are pregnant when he is prescribing medicines for you.

Effects of drugs on breastfed babies

Almost any drug present in a mother's blood will also be detectable in her milk but its concentration in the milk depends on many factors. Only a few drugs are known to cause problems — there has been surprisingly little research done in this field — and those few are here outlined:

Alcohol: A long believed fallacy is that a drink taken by the mother half an hour before a feed sedates the baby. The truth is that it sedates the mother and even if her blood alcohol level is excessive there should be no symptoms in the infant. The only exception would perhaps be if the mother was a chronic alcoholic. This is no reason to discard the drink before feeding — it does make things easier, but for the mother rather than the baby.

Aspirin: May cause a sensitisation in the baby which means an allergy later in life, but aspirin is also capable of altering the clotting ability of the child's blood and the mother is theoretically better off taking non-aspirin painkillers.

Antithyroid drugs: Without going into medical details, if you take these drugs it is advisable to ask your doctor before getting your heart set on breast feeding.

Antibiotics: Penicillin in breast milk may sensitise the baby, causing a penicillin allergy in later life. Tetracyclines theoretically could harm the baby's teeth, as they do children's. Anaemias have been linked with treatment with sulphur drugs. It is generally believed that all antibiotics are best avoided while feeding because of the possibility of changing the normal bacterial content of the baby's intestine. The presence of normal bacteria may be important to the early development of the body's systems of immunity.

Corticosteroids: Many unwanted effects could occur and any mother taking cortisone, prednisone or other drugs of a similar nature is usually advised not to consider breast feeding.

Laxatives: Laxatives taken in quantity by the mother commonly cause diarrhoea in the infant. Phenolphthalein should be avoided, but your doctor can advise you about those that are safer.

Sedatives and antiepileptic drugs: There are a few isolated cases where adverse effects in the baby are thought to be related to ingestion of large doses of these drugs.

Note: Medication of any sort in a newborn baby is inadvisable unless prescribed by a doctor because a baby's enzyme system is very immature. So steer clear of everything unless it's medically supervised — many a well-meaning parent has fatally overdosed a baby with aspirin.

SWALLOWED OBJECTS
AND CHOKING

SWALLOWED OBJECTS

Everyone at some time swallows a few things that are not intended for eating, but the worst offenders are those nine to 18 monthers, who will consume buttons, glass, bits from toys, keys, marbles, coins — anything that fits in the mouth.

Surprisingly there is rarely any trouble. Round or squarish objects such as coins, rings, buttons or marbles take an average of five days to thread their extended way from mouth to anus and pass out quite unchanged having caused no fuss in the meantime, as long as they are small.

Large coins or buttons may get stuck in the oesophagus (food pipe) or stomach and need careful observation for 10 to 12 days before surgery is resorted to. Mostly they get through somehow!

Disc or button batteries used in calculators, watches, hearing aids etc. are easily and frequently swallowed, but they mostly pass through the system in a few days with no symptoms. Although they contain a small amount of mercury this is not sufficient to cause poisoning and in the cases where problems have arisen it has been due to the battery lodging in the oesophagus. If the battery has not appeared in the stools and the child has symptoms of pain or discomfort on swallowing, vomiting or refusing food, an X-ray is needed to see if it has become stuck.

Objects with sharp points like pins, nails and needles are naturally more dangerous, but even so they rarely make their way out through the intestinal wall but are passed in the motions normally. Medical attention is most strongly advised for safety's sake, however. Long slender objects such as pencils and bobbypins are also a bit tricky

41

because with all the corners and turns involved in the path of the intestine their length may result in their getting caught side on. Once again medical attention is strongly advised to keep an eye on the progress until the object is naturally passed, usually after about six to seven days. Surgical intervention is deemed necessary after about two weeks of fruitless waiting.

So here are some general rules regarding swallowed objects:

1. If it was a small, roundish object and the child has no symptoms, see a doctor if symptoms of pain or vomiting develop but otherwise expect it to appear in the stools within a fortnight. If you are sure the object has been swallowed and it doesn't appear, an X-ray would be a good idea. Give no special foods and no laxatives.

2. If the object was sharp or long and thin, immediate medical observation is advised because the occurrence of problems, although still uncommon, is more frequent and serious. Once again, do not give cotton wool sandwiches, laxatives or anything except a normal diet.

CHOKING

When something goes "down the wrong way" into the trachea (windpipe), it is very distressing, but only occasionally is the object large or strategically placed enough to make breathing impossible.

There are two schools of thought on immediate first aid for someone choking. One school says don't do a thing, let nature cope. The other says immediately up-end the patient and slap vigorously on the back and chest. What to do then?

I don't know medically which is best, and I don't think anyone does, but I do know that I couldn't just sit by and watch my child choke without lifting a finger to help. Psychologically, to up-end and slap must surely be the only first aid method that is feasible. If the coughing and choking doesn't immediately stop, get to hospital quickly where extraction of the offending object is usually possible with a minimum of fuss and discomfort.

Peanuts are so commonly found in the windpipe, often after months of "asthma", that all paediatricians recommend that peanuts **never** be given to children under four or five years. Even then it is a good idea to make them sit while eating them, eat one at a time and chew them well. Peanuts in the windpipe have caused death in children when left undiagnosed for too long, so it's better to avoid them completely for the first few years.

Small sharp objects, like fishbones, in the throat cause coughing and gagging but are not at all dangerous because they are not obstructing breathing. If the object is firmly stuck a doctor is needed to extract it, but more often than not the explosive coughing clears the throat which may, however, be scratched so that it feels as though the object is still there.

OBJECTS PUSHED INTO EARS AND NOSE

Peas up the nose, a beetle in an ear — children manage things like this so often and mostly they present no great problem. However, do not attempt to extract an object fitting snugly in an ear — you are sure to push it in even further. You must let a doctor remove it with the right equipment.

Things in the nose may be blown out if the child is old enough to co-operate. Get him to snort as large a breath as possible out through the nose and at the height of the snort pinch off the nostril without the foreign object — after a few attempts the object usually shoots out. Younger children may need a doctor or a casualty nurse to extract a foreign body pushed a long way up into the nose.

BITES AND STINGS

It would be impossible to discuss all the bites and stings that Australians can receive from the local animal and insect population — they are so incredibly numerous.

However, recent research has shown that the pressure bandage treatment is the best first aid in most cases of bites by venomous creatures.

The Pressure Bandage Treatment

1. As soon as possible apply a firm, wide bandage over the bitten area and as much of the limb as possible, making it as tight as you would for a sprain. Do **not** remove jeans, trousers, etc., first. A crepe bandage is best, but clothing or towels torn into strips will suffice.
2. Splint the limb using sticks and keep it absolutely still.
3. Bring transport to the victim, not the reverse.
4. Do **not** remove the bandage or splint.
5. Do **not** cut the site of the bite.
6. Do **not** apply a tourniquet.
7. Do **not** wash the bitten area. This is particularly important in the case of snake bite.

SPIDERS

Red-back spider

This spider is very common but as it seldom moves when it is disturbed, attacks are infrequent. It is not aggressive and man must make contact with it before it will bite. Only the female is dangerous. Red-back spider bites have caused deaths, but probably very few and only in children. The effects are nevertheless often severe, especially after the venom has entered the circulation, within 30 minutes of the time of the bite.

Appearance: The female red-back has a round, black body, about the size of a pea, with a red spot or stripe on the back.

Symptoms:
1. An immediate mild stinging sensation mostly occurs although sometimes there is no reaction for 5 to 10 minutes.
2. A slight swelling develops with a small red or white mark.
3. An aching pain about the affected part, and sweating, will develop as the venom enters the general circulation.
4. Intense pain, nausea and vomiting, pallor and muscular weakness may develop.

Treatment:
1. As in the case of snake bite, it is not advisable to cut the wound.
2. Immediately wash the bite to remove excess venom.
3. Give small amounts of fluid to replace water lost in sweating and also to minimise kidney damage.
4. Seek medical attention as soon as possible.

There is an antivenene to the red-back's venom and should the patient's condition be serious, the doctor will use it. For mild cases it is not required.

Habits: This spider is widespread in rural and urban areas. It prefers quiet, dark and undisturbed surroundings — such as long grass, piles of wood, empty tins or any old junk. It is frequently found in outdoor toilets.

Funnel-web spider

The most dangerous funnel-web is the Sydney funnel-web, which is found only within an 80-kilometre radius of Sydney, New South Wales. Accurate statistics of the frequency of bites are not available but they are not uncommon. The funnel-web is aggressive and will defend itself and attack when disturbed, rearing itself up quite dramatically in order to strike with its fangs. There are only a dozen or so authenticated cases of human death resulting from bites and so far as is known all of these were by male spiders. Luckily male spiders are far less common than females. Casual observations suggest that the spiders wander around above the ground most frequently in late summer, but flooding of their nests by rain will cause them to seek other shelters at any time.

Funnel-webs live for several years and they have few enemies, although kookaburras will devour them voraciously if they come out into the daylight.

Appearance: The funnel-web is a large, dead black spider with thick legs and long fangs. The male has longer legs, and a smaller body, than the female.

Symptoms:
1. Pain and numbness at the site of the bite almost immediately.
2. Excessive sweating and salivation.
3. Difficulty in breathing due to pulmonary secretion pooling.
4. Rapid deterioration in the patient's condition due to shock.

Treatment:
1. Immediately apply a pressure bandage as described on page 44.
2. Take the patient to hospital as quickly as possible. Speed is essential.

Habits: The funnel-web is essentially a ground dwelling spider, living in cavities beneath stones or around dead tree roots. It does not excavate for itself but makes use of pre-existing spaces which it lines with a finely woven, dense and fabric-like web quite different from that formed by other spiders. It does not normally come out of its hole but in wet weather or if disturbed has been found wandering inside houses. Bites have occurred as a result of their taking refuge in shoes, beds, etc.

The mature spiders always live singly but concentrations can occur in very suitable habitats.

Non-poisonous spiders

Included in this group are all Australian spiders except the red-back and funnel-web. Many species cause symptoms, occasionally very painful ones, but no deaths have been recorded. If symptoms are going to appear, they will be obvious within 10 minutes.

Symptoms:
1. Slight swelling at the site of the bite.
2. Intense pain or local irritation as with ant bite or bee sting.

Treatment:
1. Wash the site immediately with water.
2. Rub with methylated spirits to detoxify any remaining venom.
3. An ice-cube held on to the bite will help to ease the pain.
4. Observe the patient for several hours for any further symptoms and seek medical attention if the condition deteriorates.
5. Antihistamines are thought to be of no use.

Habits: May occur anywhere due to the wide variety of spiders involved.

INSECTS

Ticks

A tick bite can have very severe effects if the tick is not removed. It is especially dangerous if it is attached to the head. Deaths used to occur in children, but now there is a serum for serious cases. It is impossible to distinguish dangerous ticks from those which do not cause symptoms, as they look identical. Tiny bush ticks are harmless.

Symptoms: The initial symptoms usually develop about three to four days after attachment, but this depends on the number of ticks and the reaction of the individual. Allergy to tick bite is quite well known, and may cause quite a severe and dramatic response.

1. Headache develops, particularly when the tick is present in the scalp.
2. The victim cannot read or focus the eyes properly.
3. Blurring of vision then occurs and weakness in the limbs gradually increases to paralysis after four days.

First Aid:

1. Remove the tick immediately. This is best done with a pair of fine tweezers. The tweezers should be inserted below the body of the tick, and the head and mouthpart region seized and pulled firmly sideways. Avoid pressing the tick body, in case more venom is squeezed into the tissue. The use of irritants such as kerosene and oil is not favoured.
2. An alternative method is to loop a strong thread around the tick's head and pull. There is no truth in the tale that the head will continue to live and cause problems if left in the skin. It dies as soon as it is detached from its body.
3. If symptoms are present, apply a pressure bandage (see page 44) and take the patient to hospital immediately.

Scorpions and centipedes

Australia has several species of both, none of which has caused death.

Symptoms:

1. Immediate and intense pain and local swelling.
2. Shooting pains up the limb involved. These will probably recur in a milder form for a couple of weeks after the bite occurs.

Treatment: As for non-poisonous spider bites.

Habits: Both scorpions and centipedes live out of doors and are mainly nocturnal. They may be found in rotting vegetation, under bark or rocks and all other moist places where there are small insects for them to prey upon.

Bees, hornets, wasps

These stings are very painful and no really effective treatment is available. They are not dangerous, unless the victim is allergic to the venom. Such people require medical attention urgently upon being stung, and should be encouraged to carry an emergency kit with them at all times.

Symptoms:
1. Immediate pain and some swelling.
2. Severe allergic reactions, if they are going to occur, are almost always immediate, with intensely itching weals, breathing difficulty, shock and collapse.

Treatment:
1. Scrape the sting off with a fingernail or knife blade. Do not squeeze it with the fingertips.
2. Apply an ice-cube immediately. Heat should be avoided.
3. Rest and elevation of the limb involved will reduce the pain.
4. Should the swelling be intense or the sting occur near the eyes, nose or throat medical attention is advisable.
5. Closely observe all patients with a personal or family history of allergy for at least an hour.

Ants

Although many ants inflict painful bites, none produce dangerous symptoms.

Symptoms:
1. Pain with some swelling at the site of the bite.
2. This may turn to itchiness after 24 hours.

Treatment:
1. Rub the bite with methylated spirits.
2. Hold an ice-cube on to the sting until pain eases.

Citrus beetle

These large bronze-brown beetles squirt an irritating liquid at anyone who disturbs them in their orange or lemon tree haunts.

On the skin a mild burning sensation may be felt, but in the eye intense burning and stinging are experienced. So long as the eye is washed well immediately, no problems will arise. Seek medical attention if swelling and redness persist.

Caterpillar bristle stings

The hairy caterpillar from the cutleaf moth causes a stinging reaction when the bristles pierce the skin. They are not dangerous but can be very painful.

Treatment: Rub the area well with methylated spirits and treat the irritation with an ice-cube. The pain should ease in a couple of hours. Steroid aerosol spray (or other cortisone-like cream which is available only on prescription from a doctor) is excellent for relief of symptoms.

Habits: These caterpillars live in gum trees.

SEA CREATURES

Blue-ringed octopus

The tiny beak of this miniature octopus inflicts a painless bite, but the injected venom is extremely potent and acts rapidly. There is no antivenene, and because of the rapidity with which the venom affects respiration it is unlikely that one would be of any value.

Appearance: An octopus in miniature, with blue rings on a cream to yellow background. The blue colour deepens in intensity when the creature is annoyed.

Symptoms:
1. The bite is rarely felt; at most it is like a pin-prick.
2. Within 15 to 20 minutes difficulty with breathing is obvious.
3. Death from respiratory failure within one hour.

Treatment: Immediately apply a pressure bandage (see page 44). Get to hospital straight away, giving mouth to mouth resuscitation because the breathing muscles become paralysed. Recovery occurs after six to eight hours.

Habits: These small, attractive octopuses are quite common in rock pools all along Australia's coastline.

Bluebottles

There has never been a verified death due to the sting of the bluebottle, but the effects may be severe.

Symptoms:
1. Intense and immediate pain.
2. Multiple scattered weals each about the size of a pin's head, and growing in size.
3. Some difficulty in breathing may occur in sensitive persons.
4. Weals become extremely itchy after 24 hours.

Treatment:
1. Do **not** rub with sand or a towel.
2. Immediately apply Stingose or vinegar to inactivate venom.
3. Now rub with sand or a towel to remove remaining tentacles.
4. If necessary, apply a steroid cream (cortisone, hydrocortisone, etc.) which will immediately stop the pain. (These creams are available on doctor's prescription only.)

In eye: 1. Wash out very well with a solution of weak salt and water, making sure to remove remaining tentacles.

2. Instil some steroid (cortisone, hydrocortisone, etc.) eyedrops available only on doctor's prescription — these will prevent eye damage and stop all pain.

In mouth: This should not cause any problem but if there is excessive swelling inside the mouth see a doctor.

Sea wasp

The deadly sea wasp, also called the box jellyfish, is a great problem to swimmers in the far north of Australia. It is extremely venomous, and its sting will kill, if untreated, within minutes.

Appearance: The sea wasp differs from other jellyfish in having a box-shaped body with long venomous tentacles hanging from the four corners.

Symptoms:
1. Intense and immediate pain.
2. Red weals will appear on victim's body.
3. Patient may collapse, and death can occur within a few minutes.

Treatment:
1. Do **not** rub with sand or a towel.
2. Immediately dab with vinegar or Stingose.
3. Artificial respiration may be necessary.
4. Do **not** use a tourniquet.
5. Do **not** apply a pressure bandage.
6. Take the patient to hospital straight away.

Stinging fish

The most dangerous stinging fish is the **stonefish**, found off the north coast of Australia. It is brilliantly camouflaged, looking like a piece of old coral or algae-covered rock, and is often found in shallow pools at low tide. The spines on its back can inflict agonising wounds if it is trodden on.

Other stinging fish include the **butterfly cod**, found among the coral reefs of Queensland, the **red rock cod**, the **fortescue**, the cat fish and the South Australian cobbler. The spines of these fish may cause great pain, but the sting is not dangerous.

Symptoms:
1. Immediate intense pain.
2. Collapse may occur in the case of stonefish sting.

Treatment:
For stonefish —
1. Seek medical attention immediately. A serum is available.
2. Apply cloths soaked in hot water to the wound, to relieve the pain.
For other stinging fish —
1. Bathe wound with very hot water to relieve pain.
2. Seek medical attention. The doctor will magically ease the pain by giving an infiltration of local anaesthetic around the stab wound. A tetanus injection may also be given.

REPTILES

Snake bite

Many bites do not result in venom being injected but full precautions should be taken just in case. There need not be visible signs of the bite and pain and swelling are frequently minimal. Symptoms are varied and often transient so medical attention is essential under all circumstances.

First Aid:
1. Apply a pressure bandage immediately as described on page 44.
2. Get to a hospital or doctor without delay. If possible, take the dead snake along too.

Goanna (lizard) bites

Folklore tells that goanna bites will never heal and are quite dangerous. This is not true, but all bites should be treated. Lizards are all shy creatures and will only bite if cornered. They mostly have long needle-sharp teeth and because they eat dead flesh, have a mouth full of infective bacteria. No lizards or goannas inject a venom; the danger from a bite is solely due to the infection.

Treatment: Wash the wound very well with fast-running cold water and weak hydrogen-peroxide. If the teeth have penetrated deeply causing closed puncture wounds medical attention is essential in case of tetanus, abscesses and other infections. For superficial bites, wash well and put on a dry dressing if necessary, otherwise leave open.

ANIMAL BITES

Dog Bites

The condition of the teeth of the offender is important — smooth unchipped non-carious teeth tend to cause a clean wound, but broken teeth in older dogs may cause infection.
Treatment: Clean the wound very well with running water and then wash with hydrogen-peroxide. For deep puncture wounds, and bites with dirt or material in them, medical attention is essential, as tetanus and other infections are a real possibility. For mild bites wash well and cover with a dry dressing if necessary, otherwise leave open.

Cat Bites

Because of the needle shape of cats' teeth the bites are rarely dirty but may be deep, leading to the possibility of infection with abscess formation which is extremely serious if under a fingernail or deep in a muscle.
Treatment: Wash very well with fast-running water and weak hydrogen-peroxide and keep the area open. If the tooth has penetrated deeply medical attention is essential in case of tetanus, abscesses and other formations. If the bite is mild, wash well and cover with a dry dressing if necessary, otherwise leave open.

Cat scratches

Cat scratches are rarely deep and do not often cause immediate problems but are thought to be a cause of "catscratch disease" — an infection which appears one to eight weeks after the scratch and whose main symptom is enlarged glands.
Treatment: Wash the cat scratch very well with warm soapy water immediately. Apply a dry dressing if necessary, otherwise leave open.

VETERINARY POISONING

Animals are far less discerning than children, and often consume the most extraordinary things in search of sustenance.

Only recently a nurse rang the Poisons Centre because her fox terrier had eaten 100 sleeping pills, 12 painkillers, a plaster of paris bandage and a pair of rubber gloves and then drunk some dilute copper sulphate solution. The latter caused immediate vomiting and produced most of the former! The dog was fine. That proves my theory that dogs will eat anything. A friend of mine has a two-year-old girl and a labrador. Being of a very sharing nature, the child sat down with the dog and on a "one for you — one for me" basis, they ate two months' supply of the Pill.

I felt very sorry for the owners of a show samoyed that got to a tube of paint tinter and ate, very untidily, most of the tube. The dog was O.K. but was dyed red and white till new hair grew.

Birds also get themselves into trouble and I have dealt with galahs eating toxic plants, cockatoos drinking petrol and getting chemical pneumonia, budgerigars eating mosquito coils and even a wild seabird getting into some D.D.T. powder.

The puffer fish is a particularly poisonous fish to animals and people, as is demonstrated by the following story: A keen young fisherman, aged about eight, caught several puffers and took them home for his mother to cook. He ate a couple, despite their rather poor taste, and died. The others he had caught were given to the family dog which was promptly sick, then died. The cat ate the dog's vomit and died but was also sick. A couple of hens ate the cat's vomit and they died too. A terrible story — but it is true.

Livestock are frequently poisoned by eating large quantities of unsuitable vegetation. Some die, some get sick and others are a worry because they just don't grow at all until the farmer discovers the source of the problem. Acorns are an example of this last case.

There are a few problems that come up very frequently and so warrant specific mention.

53

Snail baits: Metaldehyde, the most common ingredient in snail baits, is very toxic to dogs and poultry and must be kept away from them at all costs. It causes tremors then convulsions and frequently, death. If the animal is treated in time by the vet, however, survival is assured.

Rat poisons: These are commonly eaten by dogs and occasionally by cats but are rarely a problem unless the animal eats a little each day for a week or so. Rat poisons contain warfarin or a close derivative and after a week will cause bleeding and death but after one dose cause no problems unless a huge quantity has been ingested. I sometimes suggest some Vitamin K tablets for a week or so if a lot has been eaten, and this assures survival.

Ant poisons: These usually have a sugary base and are a common source of severe poisoning in all domestic animals. If after half an hour the animal is vomiting a lot there is nothing anybody can do except a vet, who will have an antidote available. Always be careful where you put ant poison out, and also where you store it. If you suspect that your pet has eaten any, give lots of milk and raw eggwhite immediately and then go as fast as you can to the vet.

Benzyl benzoate: Cats have a particular sensitivity to benzyl benzoate, a common ingredient in proprietary preparations of lice-killers. It is great for dogs and kids, but even dusting on a cat will cause the rapid onset of convulsions and often death.

Pesticides: When using any pesticides around the garden be careful — most are absorbed through the skin and that includes the feet of your dogs and cats. Don't leave puddles of insecticides about for them to drink — they are much smaller than you and need correspondingly less to get severe symptoms. Once the spray is dry the worst of the problem is over and the animals can be let loose in safety.

I can't offer any general advice on treatment because the animals and the poisons are so diverse that the only person who can help you is your vet. Don't forget about the animals when you have toxic chemicals, especially tablets, around the house. One gulp and a large quantity of even the most foul tasting thing can be eaten, so be careful and thoughtful.

POISON PREVENTION

The general public readily accepts the idea that careless storage and lack of supervision are the only reasons for the poisoning of children. This idea leads to excessive guilt feelings on the part of the parent, grandparent or whoever was in charge of the child at the time of the accident, and a tendency to accuse and blame on the part of the rest of the family — and it is rubbish.

Many studies have shown that, contrary to popular belief, there is no difference between storage habits, knowledge of poisons, and supervision in homes where children have been accidentally poisoned and those in which they have not. An incredible case history will demonstrate my contention. Two unwed mothers, each with five children, lived in a five-roomed house with a sister, her husband and her four children. Meals were cooked on a wood stove and kerosene with which to start the fire was kept in an old can next to the stove. All 14 children grew up in this house and at the time that one drank the kerosene there were six children under six years living there. All had the same degree of adult supervision and accessibility to the kerosene but only one child ever drank it. Why?

The difference appears to be solely with the child. In general the poisoned children are more impulsive, extroverted, energetic, resolute and full of daring. These children have more accidents of all kinds, but because a child has these traits does not mean that it will have accidents — it just might.

There is also some relationship between poisoning accidents and a disturbed family background — the unhappy child seeking attention will do anything to attract his parent. I remember one mother who complained to me that her two-year-old child had deliberately eaten one month's supply of the Pill just to annoy her! She did not realise the awful admission she had made about her own lack of communication with her child.

Now, after saying that all the care and education in the world are of no benefit in preventing accidents, I will swim with the tide of public opinion and give you all the do's and dont's, for one can't help but feel that they must be of **some** help and even if they aren't it makes us parents feel better. Child poisoning is so frequently more important to the parent than the child, who doesn't know what all the fuss is about.

Do's and dont's

Every parent of a poisoned child feels guilty and has an excuse as to why the poisoning occurred. Over the years I have gathered a list of the most common places and situations said to be responsible for the poisoning.

Don't keep strong cleaners such as oven and drain cleaner in the cupboard under the sink. By all means leave your detergent and mild disinfectants there.

Don't mix food and dangerous things like pesticides in the same cupboard. Store them very definitely apart.

Don't store poisons in food containers; this is a common cause of death in adults too.

Don't tell children that medicines are sweets or lollies — that is really asking for it.

Don't leave medicines beside a child's bed or cot within easy reach when he awakes first thing in the morning.

Do keep a close eye on the child while you're on the phone. All children resent long telephone conversations and get up to all sorts of tricks to drag you away.

Do have a couple of childproof cupboards for your specially toxic things, handy to where you use them — one in the garage, one in the kitchen and laundry and maybe even one in the bathroom. See the carpenter's drawings in this chapter for a simple method of converting an existing cupboard.

Do check the label if giving medicines at night or in a hurry. The number of children accidentally given a dose of camphorated oil or calamine lotion instead of their own medicine is incredible.

Do keep some syrup of Ipecac in the house at all times. It is invaluable when an accidental poisoning has occurred to have a bottle of this on hand — speed is so essential and the sooner the vomiting occurs the less likely the child is to get any symptoms. It is also useful for adults whenever vomiting is thought to be desirable: overdoses, eating bad food and accidental poisoning.

Do be alert to the possibility of an accident if the normal routine of your home is broken by illness, going on holidays, visitors or going visiting.

Do throw away (by flushing down the toilet) all tablets and mixtures no longer needed.

Do try to take any medicines that you need out of the sight of the child.

Do use childproof tablet bottles, if you can procure them. They are invaluable and I believe in them totally, but unfortunately my enthusiasm is not shared by many. People without children are often the stumbling block. Why should they be inconvenienced? Or so they argue.

If you have an energetic, impulsive child who loves exploring, then implementing the above measures will decrease your chances of a disaster. However, never neglect the psychological side too. In a happy house with a good relationship between brothers and sisters and parents and children problems are less likely to arise.

A childproof cupboard

The following description of a childproof cupboard has been adapted from an article by Dr J. Woolnough which appeared in *Annals of General Practice*, June 1967.

Our basic idea here is to have an ordinary cupboard which can be easily opened by an adult, but not by a small child. The "key" to this childproof cupboard is something no child has, namely an adult sized finger.

It consists of a hole in a cupboard door through which a finger reaches to release a spring catch and open the door. A child's finger cannot reach the release catch. The door closes just like any other cupboard door, in that a catch springs over a small metal stop attached to the cupboard.

For a door of a given thickness, the diameter of the hole and the distance of the hole from the catch are both critical. A hole of a diameter about 28.5 mm (1⅛ in) has its centre a critical distance away from the rear edge of a cockspur catch inside a cupboard door. This distance is about 56 mm (2¼ in) for a door 25.5 mm (1 in) thick; 60 mm (2⅜ in) for thickness of 19 mm (¾ in) or 20.5 mm (¹³/₁₆ in); or 66.5 mm (2⅝ in) for thickness of 12.5 mm (½ in) or 16 mm (⅝ in).

Tests by members of the Australian College of General Practitioners have shown that the cupboard achieved almost 100 per cent protection for children aged two, three and four years, that is, 92 per cent of the children at risk. It was also found that the smallest adult's finger could open the cupboard.

An ingenious child will no doubt try to release the catch by poking a stick through the hole — unsuccessfully, for no straight object can open the catch. It is conceivable that a curved object like the handle of a pair of pliers could do the job, so try and keep such objects well out of reach or perhaps in the cupboard itself.

Ideally, every home could have this type of door on some of its cupboards — in the kitchen, bathroom, bedroom and especially in the toolshed or garage where petrol, kerosene, garden sprays and turpentine may be stored. In the kitchen, at least one high and one low cupboard could be provided. Incidentally, bathroom cupboards faced with mirror or glass doors would of course not be suitable for this treatment.

Care should be taken not to split the timber when cutting or drilling a hole in the cupboard door. The dimensions given here are sufficient for a carpenter to follow, but must be accurately applied. The catches are available at hardware stores and are known as "cockspur" or "elbow" catches.

CARPENTER'S DIAGRAM OF CHILDPROOF CUPBOARD.

Diagram 1

Part elevation of Cupboard door

Lipped edge of door   Cupboard frame

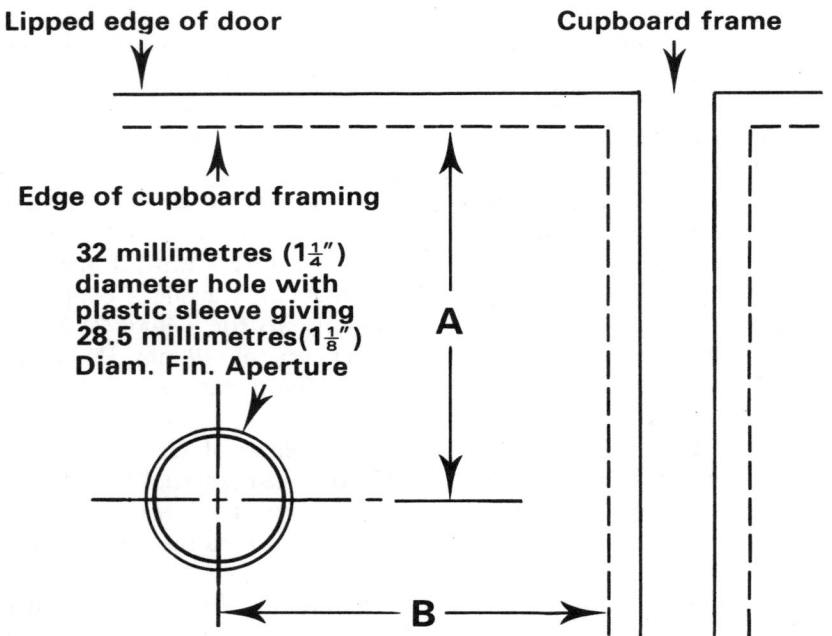

Edge of cupboard framing

32 millimetres ($1\frac{1}{4}''$)
diameter hole with
plastic sleeve giving
28.5 millimetres($1\frac{1}{8}''$)
Diam. Fin. Aperture

A

B

Diagram 2
Section through door and frame

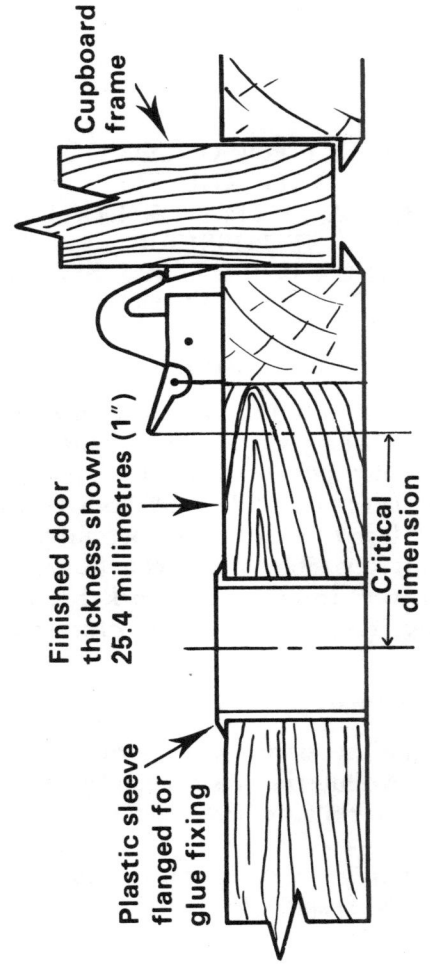

Carpenter's diagram of Child-proof Cupboard. It is desirable
that A = B, so that the catch may be fixed top or side as
required. For flush fitting doors A and B do not alter, but
position of striker should be adjusted.

FIRST AID

ACT IMMEDIATELY POISONING OCCURS — NEVER
WAIT AND SEE.
RING POISONS CENTRE OR DOCTOR FIRST
IF POSSIBLE.
ONLY MINOR POISONINGS SHOULD BE
TREATED AT HOME.

How much has been taken?

Try hard to work out **how much exactly** has been taken. If the
victim is a child, how long was he alone? What does the substance
taste like? Is there any spilt anywhere? Does the breath smell of it?
How many as a maximum could have been taken — 10, 20, 50?
Only one or two? Don't forget that a mouthful in a two-year-old is
only 3 or 4 ml, so is it possible for 200 ml to be swallowed in the time
he was alone? **It is very important to work this out straight away
before panicking. Think. Use your common sense.**

Swallowed poisons

If vomiting not necessary or desirable: Give milk, icecream or liquids to dilute the substance and give stomach a lining —
also gets rid of the awful taste. Go straight to hospital if the case is
serious.

To induce vomiting: Give **Ipecac Syrup** as soon as possible —
and go straight to the hospital if it is serious.

Ipecac dose
1 yr — 15 ml
2 yrs — 20 ml
3 yrs — 25 ml
over 3 yrs — 30 ml
adults — 50 ml

Then give a glass of **water. Repeat** dose of Ipecac and water in

20 minutes if vomiting has not occurred. This will hopefully cause a complete emptying of the stomach.

Never use Ipecac where:
(a) The patient is drowsy or unconscious.
(b) Petroleum distillates have been swallowed

e.g. Dry cleaning fluids
Fly spray (liquid)
Furniture polish (liquid)
Kerosene
Paint thinners
Petrol
Turps (mineral)

(c) Corrosive substances have been swallowed.

Note: Deaths have occurred from overdoses of the very much stronger Ipecac Tincture — make sure you have Ipecac **Syrup** — it is not possible to overdose using the above suggested doses.

If you have no Ipecac and can't get any quickly: It may be best to go straight to hospital if the case is likely to be serious. Using **salt, mustard** and other irritant substances is not only useless it is frequently **dangerous** and has caused many deaths in both children and adults.

Adults can frequently vomit by **putting a finger down their throat.** For vomiting to be useful the stomach must be emptied and if it can be induced this way give a large glass of warm water, wait a few minutes and then induce vomiting. Repeat until the stomach is empty.

It is very distressing and rarely successful to try this in children and is not recommended.

If the patient is unconscious: Go straight to hospital using blankets for warmth, giving **mouth to mouth resuscitation** if necessary (20 to 25 little puffs per minute for small children, 16 times per minute for adults). Make sure the patient is lying on his right side, **not** lying on his back, and keep the head a little lower than the body.

Poisons in the eye

No matter what splashes in the eye 10 to 15 minutes of **water** gently washing through the eye **immediately** after the incident should prevent damage. If the substance is not very poisonous then it is not necessary to keep the washing up for so long. Be very careful to wash under both lids. Do not use eyedrops unless prescribed by a doctor — the eye will fix itself up better than any eye-drop. Eyedrops are necessary for discomfort, pain or infection, but see a doctor to get them so that the extent of the problem can be assessed. Overtreating is far worse than undertreating.

Inhaled poisons

Go straight into the **fresh air** and breathe deeply.

Inhaled poisons act very quickly so if it is a serious poison such as potent insecticide get to a doctor as quickly as possible. If severe **coughing** is the problem and it doesn't improve after 10 minutes a hospital is essential — lung damage (usually reversible) may have occurred. Inhaled swimming pool chemicals will cause distressing coughing but rarely is it bad enough to need a doctor.

For the rare case of **Cyanide** poisoning do **not** inhale the exhaled air of the patient if giving resuscitation. Mouth to nose is preferable to mouth to mouth.

For the **unconscious** patient treat as outlined above under Swallowed Poisons.

POISON LIST

Toxicity rating scale (T.R.)

T.R. = 1: **Non-toxic**: Huge quantities necessary to cause symptoms.

T.R. = 2: **Slightly toxic**: Adult toxic dose about 1·136 litres (2 pints) or 908 g (2 lb). Child toxic dose about 568 ml (1 pint) or 454 g (1 lb).

T.R. = 3: **Moderately toxic**: Adult toxic dose about 284 ml ($\frac{1}{2}$ pint) or 227 g ($\frac{1}{2}$ lb). Child toxic dose about 28·4 ml (1 fl. oz) or 28·3 g (1 oz).

T.R. = 4: **Very toxic**: Adult toxic dose 28·4 ml (1 fl. oz) or 28·3 g (1 oz). Child toxic dose 1 teaspoonful.

T.R. = 5: **Extremely toxic**: Adult toxic dose $\frac{1}{2}$ teaspoonful. Child toxic dose 5 drops.

These figures assume no medical treatment. Toxic dose refers to the quantity which would cause symptoms severe enough to require treatment if the poison was not removed.

Acids

T.R. = Depends on type of acid and the concentration.

Symptoms: Immediate severe pain if it is a strong and dangerous acid. Skin is rapidly eaten away.

Treatment: On skin — wash well for several minutes and see a doctor if skin destruction is distressing. For dilute acids where no stinging or pain or skin destruction is experienced washing with water is adequate.

Swallowed — immediately give a lot of water to dilute and go straight to hospital.

See First Aid chapter (p. 60) for instructions on how to induce vomiting etc.

T.R. means Toxicity Rating scale. See p. 63

Adhesives

GENERAL PURPOSE GLUES AND PASTES
T.R. = 2–3.
Symptoms: Nil, they are usually of vegetable origin.
Treatment: Give milk.

EPOXY RESIN AND POLYSTYRENE CEMENTS
T.R. = 3.
Symptoms: May cause stinging in the mouth or allergic reactions on the skin. No burning.
Treatment: The vehicle of the glue is the problem and is not present in sufficient quantity to cause any real problem. Give milk.

After shave

T.R. = 2–3.
Symptoms: The main ingredient likely to cause a problem is alcohol, so after 20 minutes you could get signs of grogginess.
Treatment: Give milk and food to delay absorption of alcohol unless a huge quantity has been swallowed, when vomiting should be induced. Give children something sweet.

Alcohols

ETHANOL (ALCOHOLIC BEVERAGES)
T.R. = 3.
Symptoms: Ethanol is the alcohol present in alcoholic drinks and is usually what is meant by "alcohol". The symptoms are therefore those of intoxication. The stronger the drink the more alcohol present and it is possible for a child to drink a sizeable amount of a sweet drink. Young children of about one year usually have a taste for bitter things like beer. Avoid letting children have alcohol; it makes them very silly and groggy. It rarely helps them sleep.
Treatment: In young children, if the child is in a stupor take to a doctor immediately because it is possible that he could lose consciousness. If mildly affected, give lots of fluids and sweet things, as a drop in blood sugar level occurs in children. In adults, where collapse or persistent vomiting has occurred, take to hospital. Deaths

See First Aid chapter (p. 60) for instructions on how to induce vomiting etc.

T.R. means Toxicity Rating scale. See p. 63

can result from a straight alcohol overdose and usually occurs a short time after the overdose was taken.

METHANOL

T.R. = 4.

Symptoms: Vomiting and diarrhoea. A delay of up to eight hours can occur between ingestion and the appearance of symptoms. Note that methylated spirits contains little methanol.

Treatment: Medical treatment essential. Before leaving home give a large amount of an alcoholic drink, which prevents the toxic effects of methanol. If possible also give a couple of teaspoonfuls of sodium bicarbonate.

Alkalis

T.R. = Depends on the concentration and the kind of caustic.

Symptoms: Usually the symptoms are delayed five to ten minutes and then become alarmingly painful. By this time the damage is done and the tissue has been destroyed so it is important to treat immediately. There is a slimy, soapy feel to the skin.

Treatment: Swallowed — dilute with plenty of milk or water and go straight to hospital.

On skin — wash well with full strength vinegar or other available acid.

Ammonia

T.R. = Depends on concentration. In household cleaners it is never above a few per cent — T.R. = 2; in ammonia solution used for doing difficult cleaning jobs it is never above 10 per cent — T.R. = 3; in laboratory ammonia it may be as high as 28 per cent — T.R. = 5.

Symptoms: Irritation to the nose and throat, and for the higher concentrations corrosive burning of breathing passages. The symptoms are of no significance in household cleaners T.R. = 2, but T.R. = 3 cleaners could cause distressing irritation to nose, eyes, throat and lungs. The symptoms should pass off in an hour or two.

See First Aid chapter (p. 60) for instructions on how to induce vomiting etc.

T.R. means Toxicity Rating scale. See p. 63

Laboratory ammonia is dangerous, corrosive and should be treated as for strong alkalis (see ALKALIS).
Treatment: Go out into the fresh air and breathe deeply for the lower concentration preparations. If coughing is persistent and explosive then medical attention is advisable. If there is chest pain and bad coughing medical attention is essential.

Antacids

T.R. = 1.
Symptoms: Burping.
Treatment: Unnecessary.

Antibiotics

PENICILLIN
T.R. = 3.
Symptoms: May cause vomiting and diarrhoea four to 12 hours later. Severe reactions possible in those allergic to penicillin.
Treatment: None, unless there is known allergy when immediate medical attention may be either life saving or prevent uncomfortable symptoms.

ERYTHROMYCIN
T.R. = 3.
Symptoms: Usually none, but rumbles and gurgles in the stomach are sometimes reported with some vomiting, nausea and diarrhoea.
Treatment: Immediately induce vomiting if a large amount has been taken.

TETRACYCLINE
T.R. = 4.
Symptoms: Vomiting   and   diarrhoea   with   even   moderate overdose.
Treatment: Immediately induce vomiting.

Antidepressant tablets

T.R. = 5.

See First Aid chapter (p. 60) for instructions on how to induce vomiting etc.

T.R. means Toxicity Rating scale. See p. 63

Any overdose case should be immediately taken to the nearest hospital.

Antifreeze

T.R. = 4.

Symptoms: Vomiting, nausea and diarrhoea. Stinging in the mouth and throat.

Treatment: If more than 10 ml (2 teaspoons) swallowed or this is even suspected, induce vomiting immediately. If a large quantity swallowed go straight to hospital.

Antihistamines

Symptoms: Drowsiness if only a small overdose but as more are taken the symptoms change to excitation and agitation leading to prolonged and serious convulsions.

Treatment: If the patient is sleepy and drowsy let him sleep it off. If any excitability is present go straight to hospital. If you know the tablets have been taken immediate vomiting (no matter what the quantity) will prevent symptoms developing.

Antirust

FOR METALS

T.R. = 3–4.

Symptoms: Immediate stinging in the mouth and throat if the acid present is strong enough. In some preparations there are no symptoms at all. There should be no symptoms if it is spilled on the skin.

Treatment: Give large quantities of milk or icecream straight away, and if there is pain and signs of burns in the mouth, see a doctor.

FOR CLOTHING

T.R. = 5.

Symptoms: Maybe none at the time but in 24 hours if the preparation contains hydrofluoric acid, or oxalic acid, the burn could be very severe. Hydrofluoric acid causes severe skin burns

See First Aid chapter (p. 60) for instructions on how to induce vomiting etc.

T.R. means Toxicity Rating scale. See p. 63

that appear a day later.

Treatment: On skin — wash the area well and go straight to a doctor, symptoms or not, if hydrofluoric acid is involved. Hospital may not be necessary in the case of oxalic acid.

Swallowed — give milk and go immediately to hospital.

Antiseptics

T.R. = 3.

Symptoms: Usually none because the unpleasant taste discourages the taking of large doses, but if large quantities are swallowed there could be vomiting, diarrhoea and a stinging throat.

Treatment: A doctor is rarely needed because immediate vomiting occurs with the irritant undrinkable varieties. The organic mercurials (e.g. Mercurochrome) are poorly absorbed, and in one dose not a problem. Hexachlorophene in anything but enormous amounts only requires milk. Should vomiting be very severe, the antiseptic may be a less common type not covered here, and immediate medical attention is essential.

Ant killers

CONTAINING ARSENIC OR ANTIMONY

T.R. = 5.

Symptoms: Persistent vomiting after about 30 minutes followed by general collapse and shock.

Treatment: For anything more than a taste go straight to hospital after giving milk and eggwhites.

CONTAINING CHLORDECONE

T.R. = 3.

Symptoms: The containers hold so little that it is unlikely that symptoms would appear, even if the entire contents of a container was eaten.

Arsenic

T.R. = 5.

See First Aid chapter (p. 60) for instructions on how to induce vomiting etc.

T.R. means Toxicity Rating scale. See p. 63

Symptoms: Violent vomiting within 15 to 30 minutes, followed by shock.
Treatment: Give milk and eggwhites and go straight to hospital.

Aspirin

T.R. = 4.
Toxic dose for children under one year = 500 mg (2 tablets)
children of two years = 3 g (10 tablets)
Adults in excess of 10–15 g
Symptoms: Rapid, uneven breathing, ringing in the ears, then vomiting and restlessness. Symptoms may be delayed by a few hours.
Treatment: Immediately induce vomiting. Give large amounts of fluid and half a teaspoonful of bicarbonate of soda. If the toxic dose has been reached go straight to hospital, especially in the case of a child who is very sensitive to overdosing. Children can die as a result of overdosing during a period of illness. A little more than the recommended dosage, given regularly to the child for a couple of days, can result in serious illness.

Baby oil

T.R. = 1.
Symptoms: Nil.
Treatment: Nil.

Baby powder

T.R. = 1.
Symptoms: Baby powder is not poisonous, but occasionally it gets sprinkled heavily over the baby's face, and is inhaled into the lungs. This may cause a type of irritant pneumonia, so always be very careful to keep the powder out of the child's reach. If the powder is inhaled and the child is coughing badly, go to hospital in case any real respiratory difficulty should develop.
Treatment: Swallowed — no treatment necessary. Inhaled — if inhaled in any quantity, and if there is coughing and spluttering, hospital is the only answer.

See First Aid chapter (p. 60) for instructions on how to induce vomiting etc.

T.R. means Toxicity Rating scale. See p. 63

Barbiturates

Symptoms: In the first hour symptoms of release of tension may be seen before the collapse. In a child this would not occur.
Treatment: Hospital for vomiting and other suitable treatment. Most patients survive with today's excellent treatment methods.

Bath preparations (Oil, Bubbles, Salts)

T.R. = 1.
Symptoms: See Baby oil, Detergent or Salt.
Treatment: Give milk or icecream.

Batteries

See the chapter on Swallowed Objects and Choking.

Battery acid

T.R. = 3.
Symptoms: Sulphuric acid is sometimes crusted on to the outside of old batteries and can burn if touched with a moist finger or if it is licked. Sensation of severe irritation with the possibility of a blistered area on lips or tongue.
Treatment: On skin — wash well for several minutes. See a doctor if the burn is bad. In mouth — give large amounts of cold milk or icecream. See a doctor if the burn is bad.

Benzoyl peroxide

See Fibreglass Catalysts.

Bleach

T.R. = 2–3.
Symptoms: Immediate vomiting if a mouthful has been swallowed. Otherwise just sore throat and discomfort.
Treatment: Give icecream or milk to settle the stomach.

Blue

See Laundry Blue.

See First Aid chapter (p. 60) for instructions on how to induce vomiting etc.

T.R. means Toxicity Rating scale. See p. 63

Boracic acid or boric acid

See Borax.

Borax

T.R. = 4.
Symptoms: Vomiting and diarrhoea. In tiny babies the resulting dehydration is difficult to treat, and is very dangerous.
Treatment: In adults and older children, for quantities in excess of a couple of teaspoonfuls, induce vomiting. In babies, take immediately to hospital. If the baby is found within half an hour of eating the borax, give Ipecac Syrup before leaving.

Brake fluid

T.R. = 3.
Symptoms: Very irritant and so causes stinging and burning sensation in mouth and throat. Later may cause drowsiness.
Treatment: Immediately induce vomiting if more than a mouthful or two have been swallowed. Otherwise give icecream or milk.

Bromides

As for Barbiturates, except of lower toxicity.

Calamine lotion

T.R. = 1.
Symptoms: Nil, apart from a nasty taste.
Treatment: Give a glass of milk.

Camphor and camphorated oil

T.R. = 4.
Symptoms: Camphor is very rapidly absorbed and causes signs of stimulation within 15 to 30 minutes. Stimulation progresses to convulsions.
Treatment: Medical help should be sought as quickly as possible

See First Aid chapter (p. 60) for instructions on how to induce vomiting etc.

T.R. means Toxicity Rating scale. See p. 63

for all but the tiniest amounts. Give charcoal to absorb the camphor, if possible.

Carbon monoxide

T.R. = 4.
Symptoms: Headache, rapid fatigue, bad temper, nausea then obviously severe symptoms like collapse and coma.
Treatment: For mild exposure, breathing deeply in the fresh air. If the patient has been severely affected he should go immediately to hospital for oxygen therapy.

Carbon paper

T.R. = 1.
Symptoms: Nil.
Treatment: Nil.

Carbon tetrachloride

T.R. = 5.
Symptoms: These may occur after swallowing, inhalation or skin absorption and usually exhibit themselves as nausea and vomiting, drowsiness and visual difficulty.
Treatment: Fresh air and deep breathing in mild cases but hospital for all but the smallest quantities. Alcohol in the system makes carbon tetrachloride much more poisonous and small exposures regularly over several months cause hepatitis, so it is a substance to use very carefully and preferably not at all.

Carpet shampoo

T.R. = 2.
Symptoms: Stinging feeling in mouth and throat, maybe vomiting followed by diarrhoea 24 hours later.
Treatment: Lots of milk or icecream will settle the stomach.

Car polish

T.R. = 2–3.

See First Aid chapter (p. 60) for instructions on how to induce vomiting etc.

T.R. means Toxicity Rating scale. See p. 63

Symptoms: Nasty taste in the mouth, burping.
Treatment: Give milk and icecream to settle the stomach.

Caustic pencil

T.R. = 3–4.
Symptoms: Burning in the mouth.
Treatment: If only sucked, give milk, but if any quantity chewed and swallowed give orange juice or diluted vinegar (one part vinegar to 10 parts water), to neutralise it.

Caustics

See Alkalis.

Cement

T.R. = 2.

POLYSTYRENE TYPES
See Adhesives.

BUILDERS' CEMENT
Symptoms: Unpleasant taste.
Treatment: Sugar will prevent the setting of cement, though it is hard to imagine it setting rock hard in the stomach.

Chalk

T.R. = 1.
Symptoms: Nil.
Treatment: Nil.

Chest rubs

T.R. = 2.
Symptoms: Watery eyes, runny nose and awful taste — hard to eat very much.
Treatment: Give lots of icecream or milk.

See First Aid chapter (p. 60) for instructions on how to induce vomiting etc.

T.R. means Toxicity Rating scale. See p. 63

Chloral

See Barbiturates, though of lower toxicity.

Chlorine (for Pools)

T.R. = 3–4.
Symptoms: Vomiting and some local reddening and irritation if swallowed. If dust or gas inhaled, severe coughing. Reddening and irritation if comes in contact with skin or eye.
Treatment: In eye — wash out very well. No real damage should have occurred but if the eye gets angry and red see a doctor in case of infection.

Inhaled — if coughing continues after 20 minutes and is causing respiratory distress, go to hospital.

Swallowed — should not cause corrosive burning but if you suspect a severe burn have it checked by your doctor. Give milk to help settle the stomach and reduce nausea.

Cigarettes

Symptoms: Children who eat cigarettes, vomit.
Treatment: If the child has eaten more than one whole cigarette he will vomit a lot, so it is a good idea to give charcoal to prevent this distress. Your doctor may be needed if two or more cigarettes have been eaten.

Clay

See Modelling Clay.

Cleaners

Also see Drain, Oven, Metal and Toilet Bowl Cleaners.
T.R. = 2.
Symptoms: Whether powder, paste or liquid little harm but quite a degree of discomfort is likely to occur. Most cleaners are irritant but not corrosive and so cause a sore throat and a stinging mouth. Vomiting is possible. The "marvel" ingredients are never dangerous, more likely just gimmicky.

See First Aid chapter (p. 60) for instructions on how to induce vomiting etc.

T.R. means Toxicity Rating scale. See p. 63

Treatment: Give milk or icecream immediately.

Cloudy ammonia

See Ammonia.

Codeine

Symptoms: This drug is present in many cough mixtures and headache tablets. It is not very poisonous and the other ingredients present in both these types of preparations are likely to be more poisonous. Symptoms due to codeine itself are restlessness, nausea and excitability.
Treatment: Induce vomiting immediately. If symptoms are obvious seek medical advice as both cough mixtures and headache tablets contain several other ingredients, and it may be hard to determine what is causing the problem.

Coins

Symptoms: Small one or two cent coins usually go through with no problems. The metals are non-toxic.
Treatment: No laxatives, a normal diet. Should abdominal pains develop within a couple of weeks (the coin may get stuck somewhere) see a doctor and mention the episode. An X-ray will soon tell whether or not the coin is causing the pain.

Condy's crystals

T.R. = 4.
Symptoms: Only mildly irritating in dilute solutions but highly corrosive as a concentrated solution or dry crystals. Causes destruction of tissue inside the mouth which should be obvious despite the strong discoloration.
Treatment: For very dilute solutions where no symptoms of burning are felt, just give milk and raw eggwhite — I suggest an eggflip with sugar and vanilla. Otherwise a hospital is essential. See Alkalis.

See First Aid chapter (p. 60) for instructions on how to induce vomiting etc.

T.R. means Toxicity Rating scale. See p. 63

Contraceptive foams, gels, creams

Symptoms: Usually only small amounts are swallowed, resulting in no symptoms at all. Poisonous chemicals cannot be used in these products because the vagina has a very absorbent surface.
Treatment: Milk, to get rid of the taste.

Contraceptive pills

See Oral Contraceptive.

Cosmetics

T.R. = 1 — 4.
Symptoms: These are dealt with under individual headings, but in general, despite the very occasional toxic ingredient, such small quantities of these products are swallowed that poisonings never occur. Perfumes and aftershaves contain quite high concentrations of alcohol, and these are the only products likely to cause trouble.
Treatment: If you are at all worried induce vomiting immediately, although this shouldn't be necessary.

Cough mixtures

Symptoms: The range of ingredients present in cough mixtures is very wide indeed. If the mixture is a doctor's prescription it may be very dangerous and could contain a narcotic anti-coughing drug. This needs treatment for even a few mls in a child. Others that are freely available from your chemist should not be too bad in small overdoses but always check up — it's not worth risking it. Symptoms may be sedation and sleepiness or the other extreme of overexcitation and wild behaviour.
Treatment: Induce vomiting for all overdoses caught within half an hour. For overdoses of non-prescription mixtures discovered after this time, let the child sleep it off, unless he is exhibiting distressing symptoms, when medical advice should be sought. For overdoses of prescription mixtures discovered too late, seek medical advice.

See First Aid chapter (p. 60) for instructions on how to induce vomiting etc.

T.R. means Toxicity Rating scale. See p. 63

Crayons (Children's)

T.R. = 1.

Symptoms: Nil — children's crayons do not contain poisonous dyes.

Treatment: Nil.

Creosote

See Phenols.

Dandruff shampoos

See Shampoo.

Deodorants — household

BLOCKS

T.R. = 3.

Symptoms: Active ingredient is usually p-dichlorobenzene and quite a large chunk (about 20 g) must be eaten before symptoms appear. First symptoms are vomiting and diarrhoea after about 30 to 60 minutes, followed by sedation.

Treatment: If a large amount has been eaten vomiting might be a safe measure. If just a nibble or two has been taken, don't worry.

LIQUIDS

T.R. = 3–4.

Symptoms: Some contain kerosene-like liquids which are easily discernible by the smell. The label will also give this information. For these treat as for Kerosene.

The other liquids with a fresh, chlorophyllish smell are not poisonous at all.

AEROSOLS

T.R. = 1.

Symptoms: Nil unless sprayed in the eye, when irritation and reddening will occur.

Treatment: If sprayed in eye, wash well with warm water.

See First Aid chapter (p. 60) for instructions on how to induce vomiting etc.

T.R. means Toxicity Rating scale. See p. 63

Deodorants — personal

T.R. = 3.

Symptoms: Some may cause a tingling or burning feeling on the tongue but unless a whole bottle has been swallowed there should be no problem.

Treatment: For a few licks or bites or squirts from an aerosol, give milk. If a lot of the liquid preparation has been taken (highly unlikely because of the taste and burning feeling), give milk and take to hospital.

Desiccant crystals

T.R. = 1.

Symptoms: Nil. Little bags of these crystals are included with a lot of tablets and other chemicals to keep the moisture to a minimum. They are quite non-toxic, containing only silica gel.

Treatment: Nil.

Detergents

T.R. = 2.

Symptoms: Occasionally these cause vomiting and foaming at the mouth, due to the bubbles coming up. They certainly cause a sore throat and nausea in adults but children rarely complain of these. Diarrhoea may occur transiently next day.

Treatment: Lots of milk, especially if there has been any vomiting or if it looks imminent.

Disinfectants

T.R. = 3.

STANDARD DISINFECTANTS

Symptoms: As for detergents — the disinfectant ingredient is not a hazard.

Treatment: As for detergents.

STRONG PHENYLE DISINFECTANT

T.R. = 4.

See First Aid chapter (p. 60) for instructions on how to induce vomiting etc.

T.R. means Toxicity Rating scale. See p. 63

Symptoms: Burning sensation in the mouth and throat. It would be hard to swallow much by accident.
Treatment: If just a sip taken, give lots of milk and icecream and an eggflip with raw eggwhites. For a large deliberate ingestion hospital is essential, because both the liver and kidneys may be affected.

Drain cleaners

T.R. = 5.
Symptoms: Treat as for very strong corrosive alkali. The cleaner will eat the tissue very quickly causing severe chemical burns and swelling about the lips, tongue and throat.
Treatment: See Alkalis.

Dry cleaning fluids

T.R. = 3.
Symptoms: There are two main kinds, those with a kerosene-like base and those with a solvent trichlorethylene or perchlorethylene base. For the first type see Kerosene. For the second type swallowing would cause nausea and vomiting. Inhalation is more serious, causing drowsiness, dizziness and may cause loss of consciousness.
Treatment: For the white spirit-kerosene types see Kerosene. For the perchlorethylene and trichlorethylene if swallowed give lots of milk and if inhaled get the patient into the fresh air immediately. See a doctor if the patient is behaving very strangely. It is not a good idea to work with these chemicals without proper precautions. Trichlorethylene is not very toxic — it is more commonly called Trilene and is used as a gas to help women during labour.

Dyes—fabric

T.R. = 3–4.
Symptoms: It is hard to envisage a situation where a very large quantity was swallowed. The possible chemical ingredients, and the symptoms resulting from them, are too varied to specify.
Treatment: If more than just a taste or two has been taken, induce vomiting immediately and go to the hospital for a check-over.

See First Aid chapter (p. 60) for instructions on how to induce vomiting etc.

T.R. means Toxicity Rating scale. See p. 63

Eardrops

T.R. = 3.

Symptoms: The smallness of the bottle and the usual ingredients make eardrops an unlikely source of trouble. Antibiotic drops are quite safe if swallowed; earache drops may sting the mouth, but little else.

Treatment: Give milk.

Epoxy resin glues

See Adhesives.

Erythromycin

See Antibiotics.

Eyedrops

T.R. = 3.
As for Eardrops.

Felt pen ink

T.R. = 1.
Symptoms: Nil.
Treatment: Give milk.

Fertilisers and liquid manures

T.R. = 3.

Symptoms: It is hard to imagine anyone eating enough of these products to get symptoms, and these would be very mild, consisting only of nausea with the remote possibility of vomiting. Even the time-release fertiliser pills cause no problem.

Treatment: Give milk.

Fibreglass catalysts e.g. MEKP, Cyclohexanone, Benzoyl peroxide

T.R. = 4.

See First Aid chapter (p. 60) for instructions on how to induce vomiting etc.

T.R. means Toxicity Rating scale. See p. 63

Symptoms: These organic peroxides cause severe irritation and burning in the mouth and throat if swallowed and excruciating pain if spilled into the eye or ear.
Treatment: Swallowed — give milk or water immediately. For quantities over a few mls, medical advice should then be sought.
In eyes or ears — wash well with floods of water immediately. Medical attention essential.

Fireworks

T.R. = 3.
Symptoms: The ingredients present in greatest quantities — those that produce the light or the bang — can cause stomach ache with some vomiting and diarrhoea, if swallowed in fair amounts. The colours and exotic effects are occasionally more lethal, but are present in the firework in tiny concentrations. Sparklers are safe.
Treatment: If several colourful fireworks or big bungers have been eaten, induce vomiting immediately. Otherwise give milk.

Fish medications and preparations

T.R. = 2–3.
Symptoms: None. Fish are very sensitive and only mild chemicals are used for their fungus diseases, etc. Urine may become the colour of the preparation swallowed, i.e. blue or green.
Treatment: Give milk.

Floor polish

T.R. = 2–3.
Symptoms: The nasty taste makes it unlikely that much floor polish would be swallowed, but should this happen the most likely symptoms would be nausea and diarrhoea.
Treatment: Avoid vomiting by giving lots of milk and icecream.

Floor stripper

T.R. = 4.
Symptoms: These liquids contain corrosive alkalis. All the

See First Aid chapter (p. 60) for instructions on how to induce vomiting etc.

T.R. means Toxicity Rating scale. See p. 63

problems of medium-strength alkalis are likely to occur. See Alkalis.
Treatment: See Alkalis. Medical attention for a check-up is essential.

Fluoride tablets

Symptoms: Ingestion of between 50 and 150 will cause a little diarrhoea. Smaller numbers will have no effects.
Treatment: Give lots of milk and icecream.

Fly spray

AEROSOL

T.R. = 1.
Symptoms: In the eye will sting, otherwise nil.
Treatment: Swallowed — nil.
  In eye — wash well with water.
  Inhaled — take patient into fresh air and encourage to breathe deeply.

LIQUID

T.R. = 3.
Symptoms: Symptoms are due to the kerosene present, not the chemicals. See Kerosene.
Treatment: See Kerosene.

IMPREGNATED STRIPS

T.R. = 2.
Symptoms: Nausea and headache can result if too many strips are used in a room, or if the strip is licked or left in contact with the skin for about 30 minutes.
Treatment: Cease exposure and the symptoms will go within a few hours.

Furniture polish

AEROSOL

See First Aid chapter (p. 60) for instructions on how to induce vomiting etc.

T.R. means Toxicity Rating scale. See p. 63

T.R. = 1.
Symptoms: Swallowed — nil.
  In eye — stinging and irritation.
Treatment: Swallowed — give milk.
  In eye — wash well with warm water.

Garden sprays

See Garden Chemicals, First Aid Chart, p. 14.

Gas—household

See Carbon Monoxide.
  Many areas now have non-poisonous gas. A quick phone call to the gas company will tell you which sort you have.

Glass

T.R. = ?
Symptoms: Little is known about the effects of swallowing glass, although it is known that ground glass is not poisonous, even if eaten regularly. Ground diamonds are, however, very dangerous, but not many people can afford them. Small chips of glass are frequently swallowed by children and adults alike and never seem to cause any problems.
Treatment: Remove as much glass as possible from the mouth, then try to forget about the incident unless any symptoms (e.g. pain in the stomach) appear, when a medical check-up would be advisable. X-rays won't show glass, laxatives are likely to make any problem worse, and cotton wool sandwiches or other odd diets are of no proven value. You can completely relax after two or three weeks.

Glues

See Adhesives.

Golf ball centres

T.R. = 1.

See First Aid chapter (p. 60) for instructions on how to induce vomiting etc.

T.R. means Toxicity Rating scale. See p. 63

Symptoms: The solution is not poisonous. The pressure at which the solution spurts out is the problem, as this can damage the eye.
Treatment: See a doctor immediately to assess damage.

Hair dyes

T.R. = 3–4.
Symptoms: On skin — some people are very allergic to these dyes, and I would suggest you follow the manufacturer's advice and do a patch test before going ahead and putting it all over your head.

Swallowed — if more than about 10 ml of a strong dye is swallowed the person goes blue all over. The more permanent the dye the more toxic it is likely to be. .
Treatment: On skin — for the allergic swelling, go to hospital, because this can be a nasty problem.

Swallowed — if a lot of dye is swallowed induce vomiting, give milk or water, and go to hospital. If just a sip or two taken, give milk.

Hair shampoo

See Shampoo.

Hairspray

AEROSOLS
T.R. = 1.
Symptoms: Stinging, if sprayed in eye; coughing if too much is inhaled in one breath.
Treatment: In eye — wash eye well with water; there will be no damage.

Inhaled — take patient outside and encourage to breathe deeply.

LIQUID
T.R. = 2.
Symptoms: The stickiness and taste would make eating in any real quantity impossible. These liquid sprays have a little methylated spirits in them, but this is unlikely to cause a problem.
Treatment: Give milk.

See First Aid chapter (p. 60) for instructions on how to induce vomiting etc.

T.R. means Toxicity Rating scale. See p. 63

Hand and body lotions

T.R. = 2.

Symptoms: Except under the most extraordinary circumstances the only symptom likely or possible would be a little diarrhoea.

Treatment: Give milk or icecream.

Hexachlorophene

T.R. = 2.

Symptoms: Soaps and lotions occasionally still contain a little hexachlorophene, but after one dose, even of 20 to 30 ml, no symptoms would be expected. If they did occur they would be vomiting and diarrhoea.

Treatment: Induce vomiting if very large quantities taken, otherwise give milk to settle the stomach.

Hydrogen-peroxide

T.R. = 2.

Symptoms: One hundred volume peroxide stings and burns the mouth a little and has an unpleasant taste, but once it reaches the stomach it becomes oxygen and water so all that happens is a big burp. Thirty and 60 volume peroxide react similarly, but with proportionally less strength.

Treatment: Give lots of milk.

Indelible pencil

See Pencils.

Inks

MARKING INK

T.R. = 4.

Symptoms: All ingestions of marking ink should be treated seriously. The throat and mouth would be burned but also there is likely to be some aniline present which affects the blood and its ability to carry oxygen. Aniline causes the body to go very obviously blue all over, especially at the lips.

See First Aid chapter (p. 60) for instructions on how to induce vomiting etc.

T.R. means Toxicity Rating scale. See p. 63

Treatment: Induce vomiting immediately and go straight to hospital.

WRITING AND ENDORSING INK
T.R. = 2.
Symptoms: Symptoms unlikely to occur even if a whole bottle swallowed. Red ink is thought to be more of a problem than the others.
Treatment: If a lot of red ink is drunk, induce vomiting. Otherwise, give milk.

Insecticides

The variety is such that generalisation is impossible. Many insecticides are extremely toxic and far-reaching in their effects, others almost inert.

See Garden Chemicals, First Aid Chart, p. 14 for the most common. If in any doubt, ring your Poisons Information Centre, or doctor. They may need to know the exact composition of the substance in question, so have the packet or bottle with its label information handy. If symptoms are distressing and severe go straight to hospital.

Insect repellents

AEROSOL
T.R. = 1–2.
Symptoms: Stinging if sprayed in the eye. Otherwise no symptoms.
Treatment: Wash eye well.

LIQUIDS
T.R. = 3.
Symptoms: Over about 15 ml swallowed by a child may cause gastric irritation and some vomiting, but because of the really nasty taste it is very unusual for a child to swallow more than a mouthful. Drowsiness could also be expected when large quantities swallowed.
Treatment: Unless an extraordinarily large quantity has been swallowed giving milk is sufficient. Icecream is also helpful.

See First Aid chapter (p. 60) for instructions on how to induce vomiting etc.

T.R. means Toxicity Rating scale. See p. 63

Iron tablets

T.R. = 4.

Symptoms: Two tablets may cause distressing and even severe symptoms. Fourteen tablets may be lethal to a two-year-old. Vomiting and diarrhoea are the first symptoms but these may be delayed by several hours.

Treatment: If there is any chance that some iron tablets have been eaten induce vomiting immediately — never wait and see. If you are fairly sure that a lot have been swallowed induce vomiting and get to your nearest hospital with all speed.

Kerosene, turps and other petroleum distillates

T.R. = 4.

Symptoms: Trouble begins in two ways — the first and the most dangerous is when there is immediate choking coughing with breathing difficulty. This may develop very quickly to a stage where it is impossible to treat so the patient must get to a hospital as quickly as possible. This problem occurs when a lot of the petroleum distillate has gone down the wrong way into the lungs instead of the normal way to the stomach.

The second occurs when just a little goes down into the stomach and there is some coughing and maybe vomiting. This doesn't last and in no time everything seems normal. The matter may end there, but watch very carefully for three to four days. If a pain in the chest, temperature and painful coughing develop go immediately to hospital, as these may signal the onset of chemical pneumonia which needs instant attention.

Treatment: Try to give milk straight away and follow it with icecream to settle the stomach and prevent vomiting. Vomiting is likely to result in even more of the liquid getting into the lungs. If there is **any** breathing difficulty go to hospital without delay.

Laundry blue

T.R. = 1.

Symptoms: Both liquids and solids are non-toxic but may cause

See First Aid chapter (p. 60) for instructions on how to induce vomiting etc.

T.R. means Toxicity Rating scale. See p. 63

the urine to go bright blue.
Treatment: Nil.

Laxatives

Symptoms: Because they are frequently pretty coloured little tablets it is not unusual for a child to eat very large numbers. Symptoms are delayed at least four to six hours and are naturally those of colic-type pain, rumbles and grumbles and then explosive diarrhoea for up to 48 hours. This of course is most unpleasant and distressing and may cause the bottom to become very red and irritated.
Treatment: If more than a couple of tablets taken, give some anti-diarrhoea mixture to keep the pain and explosions down. If more than about 10 taken, induce vomiting immediately to prevent prolonged agony. If things become really painful a doctor can prescribe something stronger than anti-diarrhoea mixture to decrease the irritation.

Lead

T.R. = 3.
Symptoms: Symptoms of chronic long-term lead poisoning are poor appetite, vomiting and diarrhoea, crankiness and loss of weight. Although not immediately obvious, brain damage is common. Recovery is very slow and requires a lot of treatment. To be poisoned by one dose of lead is very rare indeed. A piece of lead metal needs to stay in the stomach for at least a fortnight before it will slowly begin to produce the symptoms of chronic lead poisoning, often taking months to become obvious. Lead sinkers or lead shot usually pass through the body in one to three days with no trouble.

The most common cause of lead poisoning in children is the odd habit of eating paint peeling from walls. It is necessary to eat only a few milligrams of lead, which would probably be present in a piece of paint as big as your little fingernail, each day for several months, to be affected. If more is eaten daily then symptoms appear sooner. Some children have been affected by chewing the paint from their cots while teething.
Treatment: Prevent the problem occurring in the beginning by

See First Aid chapter (p. 60) for instructions on how to induce vomiting etc.

T.R. means Toxicity Rating scale. See p. 63

stopping all paint swallowing. Strip the cot back to its natural material and scrape off the flaking paint outside. It is hard to break children of the paint-chewing habit, once they are hooked on it. If you are worried that you might have a case of lead poisoning on your hands see your local doctor immediately.

Lead pencil

T.R. = 1.
Symptoms: Nil. "Lead" pencils are made from graphite, a type of carbon, not lead.
Treatment: Nil.

Lighter fluid

T.R. = 4.
See Kerosene.

Lime

UNSLAKED LIME (QUICKLIME)
T.R. = 3.
Symptoms: Very corrosive and burning in eye or if swallowed.
Treatment: In eye — immediately wash very well with a continuous stream of water for 10 minutes to prevent the quicklime eating into the eye, then have a doctor look at the eye to make sure there has been no damage to the cornea.

Swallowed — give any liquid handy, preferably an acid such as diluted vinegar, fresh orange juice, etc. See Alkalis.

SLAKED LIME
T.R. = 1.
Symptoms: Nil. This is a very mild alkali which does not burn.
Treatment: None necessary. Milk or food will settle the stomach.

Lipstick

T.R. = 1.
Symptoms: Nil.
Treatment: Nil.

See First Aid chapter (p. 60) for instructions on how to induce vomiting etc.

T.R. means Toxicity Rating scale. See p. 63

Lozenges—throat and cough

T.R. = 1–3.

Symptoms: To exceed the recommended dosage of lozenges that have been bought without a prescription from a doctor would usually cause nausea but little else. There are a very few potent throat lozenges that are used for severe throat conditions and available only on prescription and these should be regarded as quite toxic.

Treatment: For the ordinary cough and throat lozenges, the nausea will pass, so long as the patient stops eating them. For the stronger prescription lines, induce vomiting immediately and go straight to hospital.

Lubricating oil

T.R. = 1.

Symptoms: This has an awful taste, so only a small amount would be drunk. Causes nausea.

Treatment: Give lots of cold milk or icecream to prevent vomiting occurring. Some diarrhoea may occur next day for a short period.

Makeup

T.R. = 2.

Symptoms: The only poisonous kinds of makeup are a few acne preparations and even for these a large quantity must be eaten before symptoms appear. Cleansers, foundation, powder, mascara, eye-shadow are all safe when eaten.

Treatment: For almost all, no treatment needed, for perfume, acne preparations and other astringents see Alcohol.

Match heads and boxes

T.R. = 2.

Symptoms: Match heads are not made of phosphorus but of potassium chlorate. About 60 matches need to be eaten by a two-year-old before symptoms (stomach pain and maybe some vomiting) occur. The striking surface on the matchbox is red phosphorus and is non-toxic — only white and yellow phosphorus are dangerous.

See First Aid chapter (p. 60) for instructions on how to induce vomiting etc.

T.R. means Toxicity Rating scale. See p. 63

Treatment: Give milk and icecream. This should be enough so long as no more than a boxful has been eaten. The vomiting and tummy pain are quite shortlived and should not be a worry even if lots of matches have been swallowed. If symptoms persist, however, see a doctor.

MEKP

See Fibreglass Catalysts.

Mercury

FROM THERMOMETERS
T.R. = 1.
Symptoms: Nil. Metallic mercury is quite inert.
Treatment: None necessary.

FROM MERCURIAL ANTISEPTICS
T.R. = 2.
Symptoms: These organic mercurials are poorly absorbed. About 100 ml is the toxic dose in a child, and the toxicity is mostly due to the alcohol in which the mercury is dissolved. Symptoms are likely to be those of intoxication.
Treatment: Give lots of milk or icecream. If large quantity swallowed see Alcohol.

Metal polishes and cleaners

T.R. = 3.
Symptoms: These vary greatly in composition but most are not very poisonous. All are likely to cause nausea, but for small quantities there should be no further problem.
Treatment: For small quantities, which is likely to be the case except for deliberate overdose, giving milk and icecream should be sufficient. Otherwise a medical check-up would be a good idea.

Methanol

See Alcohol.

See First Aid chapter (p. 60) for instructions on how to induce vomiting etc.

T.R. means Toxicity Rating scale. See p. 63

Methylated spirits

T.R. = 3.
Symptoms: Because it is 95 per cent pure alcohol see Alcohol.
Treatment: See Alcohol. Large quantities are rarely swallowed by children due to the unpleasant taste and smell.

Methyl ethyl ketone peroxide

See Fibreglass Catalysts.

Modelling clay

T.R. = 1.
Symptoms: None. Children's modelling clay is non-toxic.
Treatment: None necessary.

Money

See Coins.

Mosquito coils

T.R. = 1.
Symptoms: Such a small quantity is commonly eaten that no symptoms occur. A child would need to eat several full coils to get into trouble.
Treatment: None necessary.

Mothballs

T.R. = 4.
Symptoms: One does not cause symptoms, but any more than this may cause diarrhoea, vomiting and restlessness.
Treatment: Vomiting should be induced immediately if any more than two balls have been eaten.

Nail hardeners

T.R. = 3.
Symptoms: There are two types, those containing formalin (you

See First Aid chapter (p. 60) for instructions on how to induce vomiting etc.

T.R. means Toxicity Rating scale. See p. 63

can tell these by the smell) and those that have a strengthened lacquer base (which smell just like ordinary nail polish). Formalin is very irritant and causes vomiting and a burning sensation in the mouth. Lacquer is also irritating and may cause a stinging feeling. For this reason neither of the two is likely to be swallowed in any quantity.

Treatment: Give milk or icecream if less than about 20 ml has been taken. If more than this has been swallowed, induce vomiting.

Nail polish

T.R. = 2.
Symptoms: None. The colour is made from insoluble non-toxic pigments and the lacquer is not toxic.
Treatment: Give milk.

Nail polish remover

T.R. = 3.
Symptoms: A burning sensation in the mouth occurs immediately so only a small quantity is likely to be swallowed. Larger amounts will cause drowsiness.
Treatment: For small quantities, give milk and icecream. If very large amounts have been swallowed, induce vomiting.

Naphthalene

See Mothballs.

Nappy rinses

T.R. = 4.
Symptoms: Immediate vomiting if any sizeable quantity has been swallowed, otherwise mild nausea.
Treatment: Give a little bit of ordinary hand soap dissolved in water and mixed with cordial. This will inactivate the toxic ingredient. Then give lots of milk.

See First Aid chapter (p. 60) for instructions on how to induce vomiting etc.

T.R. means Toxicity Rating scale. See p. 63

Nappy washes

T.R. = 3.

Symptoms: Nappy washes contain a mixture of bleach and detergent and therefore are irritating in the mouth and taste awful. Because they are powders it is difficult to imagine a child eating a great quantity. There may be a little diarrhoea next day.

Treatment: Give milk or icecream. This should be sufficient, but if vomiting persists, see a doctor.

Oil

See Lubricating Oil (this includes Sump Oil).

Oral contraceptives

T.R. = 2.

Symptoms: Most children get nauseous and vomit after twelve or so hours, and don't feel like eating, if they swallow a few, but even one month's supply should cause no problem apart from this.

Treatment: If two to three months' supply taken at once, induce vomiting just to be on the safe side.

Oven cleaners

T.R. = 5.

Symptoms: See Alkalis, due to the very high proportion of caustic present in these products.

Treatment: See Alkalis.

Paints

ARTISTS' OIL

T.R. = 3–5.

Symptoms: Rarely any immediate symptoms. Possibility of nausea, vomiting and diarrhoea.

Treatment: Some of these paints are quite safe but others may contain lead, mercury and arsenic so it is essential to induce vomiting if quantities larger than just a lick or two have been taken.

HOUSE PAINT

T.R. = 3.

See First Aid chapter (p. 60) for instructions on how to induce vomiting etc.

T.R. means Toxicity Rating scale. See p. 63

Symptoms: Water-washable paints will not cause symptoms. Oil-based paints are likely to cause a little stinging in the mouth. Treatment: Giving milk should be sufficient. Vaseline is useful for removing oil-based paint from delicate skin where turps would be too severe.

CHILDREN'S PAINTS

T.R. = 1.
Symptoms: Australia, U.K. and U.S.A. require all children's paints to be non-toxic, so no symptoms will occur.
Treatment: None necessary.

Paracetamol

Symptoms: In small doses (less than 2 g in a two-year-old or 10 g in an adult) no symptoms occur, but in higher doses all sorts of problems arise, two to three days later when the liver ceases to function normally and nausea, jaundice and general illness result. So if the patient doesn't develop symptoms immediately don't automatically conclude that all is well.
Treatment: If there is even the remotest possibility that the abovementioned quantities or more have been swallowed, induce vomiting immediately and seek medical attention.

Paste

See Adhesives.

Pencils

T.R. = 1.
Symptoms: None. Indelible pencils, coloured pencils and ordinary lead pencils are not poisonous.
Treatment: None necessary.

Penicillin

See Antibiotics.

See First Aid chapter (p. 60) for instructions on how to induce vomiting etc.

T.R. means Toxicity Rating scale. See p. 63

Perchlorethylene

See Dry Cleaning Fluids.

Perfume

T.R. = 2–3.

Symptoms: The toxicity of skin perfume is due to the alcohol present which may be from 10 to 60 per cent depending on the price of the product. See Alcohol for quantities over 10 to 20 ml. Concentrated perfumes are more poisonous but usually are in small bottles with a tiny hole at the top so large ingestions are very rare. They cause immediate and persistent vomiting.

Treatment: Skin perfumes — give food, milk and icecream for small quantities. See Alcohol for larger amounts. For concentrated perfumes — give milk for a small amount, but see a doctor immediately if vomiting is persistent.

Peroxide

See Hydrogen-peroxide or Benzoyl Peroxide.

Pesticides

See Garden Chemicals, First Aid Chart, p. 14.

Pest strips

See Fly Sprays.

Petroleum distillates

See Kerosene.

PETROL

See Kerosene.

Phenacetin

See Paracetamol.

See First Aid chapter (p. 60) for instructions on how to induce vomiting etc.

T.R. means Toxicity Rating scale. See p. 63

Phenols

T.R. = 4–5.

Symptoms: Phenolic disinfectants are little used today and are only available in a dilute non-poisonous form. Creosote is very irritant to the skin but not strong enough to be a danger. Swallowing phenolic disinfectants will cause stinging and burning in the mouth and throat. Should pure phenol or a strong solution of phenol be swallowed, medical attention should be sought immediately. The skin is also irritated by all phenols so always wear gloves and wash well if any is spilt.

Treatment: Swallowed — give lots of milk, icecream or other fatty food to protect the stomach. See a doctor immediately if a lot has been swallowed, or in the case of concentrated phenol. On skin — wash well immediately and rub in lanoline, face cream or other oily substance.

Pholcodeine

T.R. = 3.

Symptoms: This cough mixture ingredient is not very poisonous and even after swallowing 50 to 60 mg most two-year-olds only feel sleepy. If very large quantities have been taken restlessness and excitation may occur, but this is very rare.

Treatment: For quantities over 60 mg induce vomiting. Medical attention is essential for quantities over 100 mg although symptoms do occur with smaller doses.

Phosphorus—white and yellow

T.R. = 5.

Symptoms: If swallowed, inhaled or spilled on skin white and yellow phosphorus will burn severely. Red phosphorus, as is present on the striking surface of matchboxes, is non-toxic.

Treatment: Swallowed — give milk and eggwhites if handy. Rush to hospital.

Inhaled — rush to hospital.

On skin — wash with anything handy. Rush to hospital.

See First Aid chapter (p. 60) for instructions on how to induce vomiting etc.

T.R. means Toxicity Rating scale. See p. 63

Photographic chemicals

T.R. = 1-4.
Symptoms: There are few very poisonous photographic chemicals. The larger companies all put the toxic ingredients on the label and also give first aid instructions. The full formulas are never divulged.
Treatment: Follow the instructions on the label. If a great deal (say 20 ml) has been swallowed vomiting would be desirable, whatever the label instructions say. Otherwise give milk or icecream to settle the stomach.

Plants

See Poisonous Plants chapter, where plants are listed alphabetically.

Polishes

See Floor Polish, Furniture Polish, Metal Polish, Nail Polish, Shoe Polish.

Polystyrene cements

See Adhesives.

Powder

See Baby Powder.

Putty

T.R. = 1-2.
Symptoms: Mild nausea is possible, otherwise no symptoms.
Treatment: None necessary.

Quicklime

See Lime.

Radiator cleaner

T.R. = 4.
Symptoms: Usually corrosive and containing kerosene so it burns the mouth and may cause severe coughing or vomiting.
Treatment: Give milk. Do **not** induce vomiting. Go straight to hospital.

See First Aid chapter (p. 60) for instructions on how to induce vomiting etc.

T.R. means Toxicity Rating scale. See p. 63

Rat poison

T.R. = ·1–2.

Symptoms: Bleeding, from gums and scratches and sores first, then generally, will occur if small amounts have been eaten for four to seven days in a row. No symptoms will result from one ingestion, even quite large. This applies to rats as well as to people and domestic pets. It is said to be possible for a dog or cat to die after eating a whole packet of rat poison at one sitting, but I have never seen such a case.

Treatment: No treatment is necessary for a single dose. Seek medical attention immediately if it is discovered that the poison has been eaten regularly, or if bleeding occurs.

Room deodorants

See Deodorants.

Rust converter or preventative

T.R. = 3–4.

Symptoms: Preparations vary but are frequently quite strongly acidic and may cause burning in the mouth and throat. If no distress is shown by the child it is almost certain that only a tiny bit has been tasted or that the preparation is a mild one.

Treatment: Dilute immediately with enormous quantities of milk or water, or whatever is handy. If there is any persistent distress see a doctor immediately, to check for any deep burns.

Rust remover

See Antirust.

Salt

T.R. = 3.

Symptoms: The use of salt and water to induce vomiting has caused many deaths. Vomiting and diarrhoea may become very severe after some delay.

Treatment: Give the patient as much fluid as possible and take to hospital.

See First Aid chapter (p. 60) for instructions on how to induce vomiting etc.

T.R. means Toxicity Rating scale. See p. 63

Salicylates

See Aspirin. Salicylates as a general heading include methyl salicylate, salicylamide, salicylic acid and acetyl salicylic acid (aspirin).

Sedatives

For example Valium, Serepax.

Symptoms: Symptoms of euphoria, dizziness, hilarity, falling over, overactivity alternating with sleepiness and just drowsiness may occur. Unconsciousness will result from a large overdose.

Treatment: If the overdose involves a healthy person, one drug only, no alcohol and only four or five times the normal dose it can be slept off safely. Do not try to keep the patient awake by walking the floor or giving him black coffee. Restful sleep is by far the best cure. If there is any question of a large overdose, plus a lot of alcohol or several other sedative drugs, medical attention is essential. Never keep an unconscious patient (that is, one who can't be woken) at home — too many problems may arise without your knowledge. Problems include: inadequate breathing causing brain damage, low blood pressure causing kidney and brain damage, vomiting while unconscious and inhaling the vomit (often fatal), bed sores, and, the most common, catching pneumonia. See Deliberate Sedative Overdose (p. 36–37) for more details.

Shampoo

T.R. = 2–3.

Symptoms: As for Detergents except in the case of special medicated shampoos, where extra precautions are always on the label. Even the strongest medicated shampoos are rarely a problem. A two-year-old would have to swallow about 20 ml before medical attention was necessary. Too frequent washing with medicated shampoo is more often a source of trouble.

Treatment: Give milk. See Detergents for extra details. Medicated shampoos — give milk, and then vomiting may safely be induced with Ipecac if the quantity ingested is 20 ml or more.

Shaving cream

T.R. = 2–3.

Symptoms: Things may be a bit soapy, but no symptoms of any severity will occur.

Treatment: Give milk or icecream.

See First Aid chapter (p. 60) for instructions on how to induce vomiting etc.

T.R. means Toxicity Rating scale. See p. 63

Shoe polish

T.R. = 4.

Symptoms: Theoretically more than about a teaspoonful should cause symptoms in a child but I have never heard of a case of poisoning. I think the mess made encourages one to think that more has been swallowed than actually has. Symptoms would be vomiting and nausea and the rare possibility of the skin's taking on a bluish tinge.

Treatment: Give milk or icecream. If you are fairly sure that more than a full teaspoon has been swallowed, then use Ipecac to induce vomiting, just to be on the safe side.

Silica gel

See Desiccant Crystals.

Silver polish

See Metal Polishes and Cleaners.

Skin care products

See Cosmetics.

Slaked lime

See Lime.

Sleeping pills

See Sedatives, the same general rules apply.

Soap and soap powders

T.R. = 2–3.

Symptoms: Because of the irritating effect on the mouth, throat and stomach, discomfort and maybe vomiting and diarrhoea will occur. Inhaled soap powder causes explosive coughing.

Treatment: Swallowed — give milk or icecream.

Inhaled — seek medical help if the coughing continues after 10 minutes, and is still distressing.

See First Aid chapter (p. 60) for instructions on how to induce vomiting etc.

T.R. means Toxicity Rating scale. See p. 63

Snail killers

T.R. = 2.

Symptoms: Most snail killers contain metaldehyde in a very low concentration, and unless an enormous quantity is eaten, no problems should occur. There are a couple of new products now on the market which contain other ingredients, but these also cause no symptoms unless about half a packet is eaten. Caution here is suggested for dogs and poultry, which are very likely to eat large enough amounts to cause convulsions and death.

Treatment: Humans — induce vomiting if more than half a packet has been eaten.

Dogs and poultry — give any sedative you have at about the dose suggested for a human being of the same size. See a vet if convulsions develop.

Sterilising solutions for baby bottles

T.R. = 2.

Symptoms: Mild irritation in the mouth.

Treatment: Give a glass of milk to soothe the irritated areas.

Sump oil

See Lubricating Oil.

Swimming pool chemicals

DIATOMACEOUS EARTH

T.R. = 1.

Symptoms: Nil.

Treatment: Nil.

HYDROCHLORIC OR MURIATIC ACID

T.R. = 5.

See Acids.

CHLORINE

T.R. = 4.

Symptoms: Whether pool chlorine is swallowed, inhaled or

See First Aid chapter (p. 60) for instructions on how to induce vomiting etc.

T.R. means Toxicity Rating scale. See p. 63

splashed into the eyes, the main problem is always the strong irritation that it will cause — superficially burning the nose, mouth, throat and lungs. This will lead to coughing, sneezing and stinging. It will not cause serious damage, just 10 to 15 minutes of distress.
Treatment: Swallowed — give lots of milk and icecream.

Inhaled — move patient into the fresh air, and encourage to breathe deeply. If the coughing is explosive, painful and continues for longer than 10 to 15 minutes in a way that makes breathing difficult, go straight to hospital (this is a very rare occurrence).

In eye — damage is unlikely as long as the eye is washed carefully and immediately, especially under the eyelid, but see your doctor to make quite sure.

Talcum powder

See Baby Powder.

Tetracyclines

See Antibiotics.

Thermometers

T.R. = 1.
Symptoms: The mercury is non-toxic and the glass never seems to cause problems (see Swallowed Objects chapter). Other thermometers contain a variety of coloured liquids but all are present in very small quantities and are not toxic enough to cause any problems.
Treatment: Give lots of milk to get rid of the awful taste.

Toadstools

T.R. = 1-4.
Symptoms: Many varieties of toadstool are not poisonous at all, but there are some which cause symptoms. These may be severe vomiting and diarrhoea, or hilarity and hallucinations, occurring within a couple of hours of the ingestion. See Toadstools in Poisonous Plants chapter for further information.
Treatment: Seek medical attention.

See First Aid chapter (p. 60) for instructions on how to induce vomiting etc.

T.R. means Toxicity Rating scale. See p. 63

Tobacco

See Cigarettes.

Toilet bowl cleaners

T.R. = 2–4.

Symptoms: If the label states that the product contains phosphate, sulphate or bisulphite it may cause minor burns and irritation in the mouth. Other products contain disinfectants and soaps in low concentrations and at worst cause a little vomiting and transient diarrhoea.

Treatment: Phosphate, sulphate or bisulphite preparations — immediately give large quantities of milk or icecream to dilute the acid. Unless there are obviously badly burnt areas on the tongue and lips, medical attention should not be necessary.

NEVER MIX ACID TOILET BOWL CLEANERS WITH BLEACH — the chlorine gas released may be concentrated enough to kill you; it has happened.

Products containing disinfectants and soaps — give milk and icecream.

Tranquillisers

See Sedatives.

Trichlorethylene

See Dry Cleaning Fluids.

Turpentine —mineral

See Kerosene.

Unslaked lime

See Lime.

Upholstery cleaners

T.R. = 3.

Symptoms: These all contain soaps that are not very much stronger than ordinary detergent. May therefore cause some ir-

See First Aid chapter (p. 60) for instructions on how to induce vomiting etc.

T.R. means Toxicity Rating scale. See p. 63

ritation to the mouth and throat, and diarrhoea in 24 hours.
Treatment: Give milk and icecream to settle the stomach and give it a protective lining.

Vitamins

T.R. = 2.
Symptoms: Vitamin A and Vitamin D are toxic in very high doses or if given in excess of the recommended dose over a period of time. Vitamins B and C do not cause problems, no matter how many are taken. Multivitamin liquids for children are safe and cause no symptoms except the Vitamin B smell in the urine no matter how much is drunk. Hundreds of capsules would be required to poison a child.
Treatment: A whole bottle of infant vitamin liquid or drops causes no trouble so no treatment is necessary. For Vitamin A and D capsules eaten in overdose, immediately induce vomiting and seek medical attention. Never give Vitamins A and D freely or without medical supervision.

Weedkillers

These vary widely in toxicity. Never use Paraquat or Dinoc without full recognition of their potential dangers. For the rest, local irritation and skin sensitivity are possible, but always read the labels and adhere to them religiously. If a poisoning occurs check up with your local Poisons Information Centre, Department of Agriculture or hospital. See Garden Chemicals Chart, p. 15.

White spirit

See Kerosene.

Wood stains and oils

T.R. = 4.
Symptoms and Treatment: These are usually in a petroleum distillate base and the pigment is of no consequence. See Kerosene.

See First Aid chapter (p. 60) for instructions on how to induce vomiting etc.

T.R. means Toxicity Rating scale. See p. 63

Zinc cream

T.R. = 1.
Symptoms: Nil.
Treatment: None necessary.

See First Aid chapter (p. 60) for instructions on how to induce vomiting etc.

INDEX